POWERFUL MEDICINE: VITAMIN D
Shedding Light on a Worldwide Health Crisis

By: Lucinda Messer, N.D.

with Sidse Powell

Illustrated by Riley Dickens

Marcus!
Thank you so very much
for your friendship - you are
one amazing soul that I
am forever grateful to know.
Love Stac

<u>Disclaimer</u>

This book is intended to be used in conjunction with a regular treatment program through your licensed physician. It is in no way a replacement for medical advice or treatment for any condition, including vitamin D deficiency.

First published by Dog Ear Publishing
4010 W. 86th Street, Ste H
Indianapolis, IN 46268
www.dogearpublishing.net

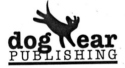

ISBN: 978-160844-327-7

This book is printed on acid-free paper.

Printed in the United States of America

To Shanti, Brian, Iva, Arrow, Corrine, Josh and Kera,
for all your loving support.

Contents

Forward

Sometimes my students make me so proud—maturing from eager learners in the classroom to vital resources for the health of our community. Dr. Lucinda Messer is such a graduate who has written a remarkable book on vitamin D.

Rarely can I say that a single nutrient is so critical to so many people's health. Although I have been studying nutrition for almost 40 years now, I had not realized the surprising importance of vitamin D until just the last few years. My awareness of the prevalence of vitamin D deficiency started with a female patient who had gone through menopause with no symptoms whatsoever. This was not surprising to me as she was living as health a lifestyle as I knew how to prescribe—organic vegetarian diet supplemented with wild caught fish, regular strengthening weight training, good supplement regime—she was doing everything right. To my great surprise a DEXA screening (an x-ray that measures bone density) showed that she was losing bone. I upped her vitamin D to 1,000 IU a day (2.5 times the RDA) and 1,500 mg of calcium—and she kept losing bone. During this time, I learned about genomic testing and had her checked. Turns out she had a genomic variation in her vitamin D receptor sites that resulted not only in difficulty absorbing vitamin D but also difficulty utilizing it effectively. As her mother and all women in her family had suffered significant osteoporosis and several had developed breast cancer, including her mother, in retrospect this was not surprising. We then increased her vitamin D to 2,000 units a day—but her DEXA showed she was continuing to lose bone and measurement of her vitamin D blood levels showed no change. So we continued to increase her daily vitamin D consumption until we hit a very surprising 10,000 iu/day. Finally, her blood levels became normal and the DEXA test showed she was recalcifying her bone. Quite an eye-opener to find that a dosage of 25 times the RDA was necessary for this woman's health! After this experience I started reading all the research I could find on vitamin D.

My learning on vitamin D took the next step when I had the opportunity to design a wellness program for a large corporation. Now being highly sensitized to vitamin D, this is one of the tests I recommended. We found that 84% of the employees were deficient and some were extremely low!

As part of the process, all of us involved in the project also had our vitamin D levels checked. Despite my taking at least 1,000 IU of vitamin D every-day and being a sun addict (yes, even in Seattle) I was stunned to find that my vitamin D was also low. After repeated blood tests at various dosages I learned that I personally have to take 4,000 IU per day during the winter to maintain healthy levels. Clearly the RDA for vitamin D is grossly inade-quate and many people in North America suffer unnecessary disease because of a deficiency in this important nutrient.

Powerful Medicine is the book I would have written if I had the time. Con-gratulations Dr. Messer and Ms. Powell for this extremely important guide to the critical importance of vitamin D for the health of everyone.

Joseph Pizzorno, ND
Co-Author *Encyclopedia of Natural Medicine*
Editor-in-Chief, *Integrative Medicine, A Clinician's Journal*
Founder, Bastyr University

Acknowledgements

This book is dedicated to the hundreds of thousands of people who have endured and suffered from vague, obscure diseases, debilitating life long diseases, terminal disease like cancer, and to anyone whose life ended much too soon and to the families they left behind.

Approximately 1 billion people in the world do not have enough vitamin D in their bodies and their health suffers greatly. And while vitamin D is not a cure-all, it is an incredibly invaluable component in our bodies and works like nothing else to keep our health in balance.

This book would not be possible without the tireless efforts of the brilliant vitamin D researches who have persisted in their work to elucidate the inner workings of vitamin D and its critical role in the optimal functioning of our bodies. Specifically, I would like to acknowledge the courageous, pioneering work of Dr. Holick, who not only published his scientific research, but who wrote a brilliant book for the general public on the importance of vitamin D. His book, *The UV Advantage,* flew in the face of big corporations who could not profit from sunshine.

I also want to thank Dr. Cannell and his colleagues at The Vitamin D Council (www.vitamindcoucil.org), who comprise the worlds leading vitamin D researchers. These genius minded researchers formed the web-based Vitamin D Council because they knew that providing their scientific knowledge to the general public could potentially have a profound impact on worldwide health.

And lastly, after working for almost two years to get this book in the hands of so many who need its guidance and information, I hope you find it to be a valuable tool in your path to health and vitality.

Sincerely,

Dr. Lucinda Messer

Chapter 1: A Health Crisis Defined

"One billion people worldwide are vitamin D insufficient."

Professor Roger Bouillon, University of Leuven

Over the past decade, treating patients in my medical practice convinced me of the importance to write a book on vitamin D and its enormous role in our health.   Unfortunately, serious and sometimes fatal health ramifications occur when vitamin D deficiency is prolonged. Vitamin D deficiency is indirectly responsible for hundreds of thousands of premature deaths worldwide. This alone imparts a great urgency to inform the public. But what is equally important, is the fact that this crisis will recess as everyone actively increases their vitamin D levels. We evolved in the sun; we were meant to have its life giving force.

We didn't always know that vitamin D was a critical player in preventing and tackling disease. But, over the past 40 years, numerous scientific breakthroughs have illuminated the vast array of mechanisms vitamin D has on our body. The past 10 years have been especially important, as vitamin D's anti-cancer properties came to light.   For the most part, this knowledge has stayed in scientific circles, and the majority of physicians remained uninformed of its far reaching effects. For instance, vitamin D was most notably known for its role in calcium regulation and bone health. What is now known and what doctors are finally learning is that vitamin D acts directly on more than 200 genes in our body. The myriad of factors that lead us toward vitamin D deficiency and the subsequent illnesses and diseases that ensued, are the main reason we now face a worldwide health crisis.

My personal experience

My understanding of vitamin D's role began over 20 years ago when I first moved to the beautiful, lush and rainy Pacific Northwest. I had been accepted into the nation's prestigious Bastyr University in Seattle and I came with an insatiable passion to understand the body and improve public health - naturally.

In medical school my energy and mood were sinking. I had grown up in the warmth of the Arizona desert and I found myself missing the sunshine and heat. I was experiencing a major shift in my mental outlook and over-all sense of well-being. Was I simply homesick? Were my studies and the pressure of medical school to blame? I started going to the tanning salon a few times a week to get a dose of sunshine and I remarkably started to feel better.

After graduating with my doctorate in Naturopathic Medicine, I returned to the Southwest where I joined a medical practice for the next three years. My first hand experience working with patients who get plenty of sunshine year round has become an important factor as I pieced together this vitamin D deficiency puzzle. The health of these patients stood out in stark contrast to me after I moved back to Seattle and opened my medical practice.

I couldn't believe how many people were sick. It was baffling. And it wasn't just my patients. Local media reports and word of mouth were always spreading news of the next bug going around, and often staying around. Everyone got sick here, and not just with the cold or flu.

I was concerned by the number of cases I was seeing of breast cancer, lung cancer, ovarian cancer, prostate cancer, MS, depression, diabetes, osteopenia, osteoporosis...the list goes on. And the numbers weren't the only startling thing; it was also the young age at which patients were being diagnosed.

My original thought was that it was because of all the rain and dense cloud cover. We weren't getting enough sunlight and I knew it. As a naturopathic doctor I was already aware that the incidence of MS is higher in the Pacific Northwest than many other places (www.whyhere.org). I also knew that MS, breast cancer and osteoporosis were not merely defi-ciencies of the pharmaceutical drugs that treat them, but rather symp-toms of a deeper pathology, namely a nutritional one in nature.

Keeping nature in mind and my awareness of the importance of sunshine, I started to ask questions. Each question leading to more and more ques-tions and finally to uncovering what is a very real, dangerous and poten-tially fatal consequence of having a vitamin D deficiency.

Could there be a common underlying link associated with the increase in disease and decrease in the age at which people are being diagnosed?

Does the exposure of sun on our skin, which is the largest organ of our body, make that much difference with acquiring disease?

Does exposure to the sun enhance our mental outlook, help us with our sleep cycles (circadian rhythms) and destroy viruses?

Have we not been told the whole truth; that we might indeed require sunlight for neurotransmitter production, immune regulation, cancer control and anti-inflammatory effects?

As health conscious individuals and parents who lather sunscreen on ourselves and our children before we step outside- are we unknowingly participating in the development and progression of life threatening diseases?

And, if sunlight is so important, how do Eskimo's fair so well in the most Northern regions of the Earth?

Yes, yes, yes, yes and yes. To answer the last question, Eskimo's have a two-fold benefit. First, they eat a diet rich in oily fish which contains one of the few food sources of vitamin D. Secondly, they live on snow covered ground for a major part of the year which reflects sunlight and increases the concentration of the UVB rays available for vitamin D synthesis in the skin.

I was now critically aware that not only does spending time in the sun give us a brighter outlook and nourish our bones, but it's also a major player in preventing disease. The lack of sunshine, whether it's due to higher latitudes, cloudy days and polluted air, or simply because our skin is soaked in sunscreen or covered in clothing, is a major reason we have epidemic cases of cancer and auto-immune diseases all over the world.

Vitamin D deficiency: A relatively new phenomenon

It wasn't until the industrial revolution that vitamin D deficiency began to have staggering effects on society with epidemic cases of vitamin D deficiency being documented. It was the turn of the century and all across Northern Europe and the Northeastern United States, 80% of children in industrialized cities were becoming crippled with Rickets, a serious bone deforming disease. This epidemic occurred specifically because a propensity for vitamin D deficiency already existed. First off, everyone living at northern latitudes are subject to a longer "vitamin D winter".

A 'vitamin D winter' is a period of months every year where vitamin D synthesis in the skin is not possible. Because of the greater distance the sun rays must travel to reach the earths surface they are virtually ineffective at synthesizing vitamin D.

Secondly, dietary sources of vitamin D are naturally scarce. The situation reached critical mass in industrialized cities where highly polluted air absorbed virtually all the useful sunlight. Without the life giving UVB rays in sunlight, children were unable to synthesize vitamin D in their skin. Without vitamin D, their bones did not form properly and the children became crippled.

Vitamin D sufficiency prevents rickets

Awareness of vitamin D's role in preventing rickets then lead to it's fortification in foods. Improvement in bone health was on the rise until the late 1940's when an outbreak of vitamin D intoxication occurred, due to poor quality control in the manufacturing process. As a result, Europe and the United States passed laws banning the fortification of vitamin D in most food products. These laws remain in effect and continue to limit our dietary sources of vitamin D.

Research illuminates vitamin D's powerful effect on the body

In the 1970's researchers began finding numerous health benefits in addition to the well documented relationship between vitamin D and bone health. Over the last 40 years, and hundreds of research articles later, vitamin D has become well known in scientific circles as a critical component for preventing life threatening diseases. The sunshine vitamin is now known to have significant effects on the immune system as an anti-inflammatory, on cellular differentiation for preventing abnormal cell growth and on inhibiting the growth of tumors.

In 1995, Dr. Mike Holick, the leading expert on vitamin D published a book called *The UV Advantage*. With the hopes of raising public awareness, Dr. Holick's work outlined the miraculous health imparting qualities of vitamin D and the serious health consequences which occur from its deficiency. His extensive research and writings on vitamin D lead him to be heralded by his peers. Yet, at the same time he was attacked politically by sunscreen companies who attempted to discredit him.

Dr. Holick is known in scientific circles as the founding father of 'The Sunshine Vitamin'. And thanks to him and the perseverance of many other researchers, we now have the groundwork of priceless information on vitamin D. There now exists years of research documenting the link between skyrocketing increases in breast, ovarian, colon, prostate and other cancers, as well as MS and a number of auto-immune diseases and vitamin D deficiency. The overwhelming evidence that lack of sunshine is the culprit keeping us ill can no longer be denied.

Why didn't I know this before?

I hear this same question from my patients. "Dr. Messer, if you're telling me that there exists 40 years of compounding, indisputable evidence of vitamin D's critical role on our health, why am I only hearing about it now?" It's an important question and the quick and simple answer is that sunshine is free. I'm not alone in believing that if a new drug held the same healing qualities as vitamin D it would be worldwide front page news. The politics of sunshine however, are complicated – just like all politics -and I've devoted an entire chapter to provide you with a look behind the scenes.

Your body: A powerful healing machine

Now before you delve into this book and gain a thorough understanding of the benefits of vitamin D, I believe it's helpful for you to know the basic truths about the human body. Being a naturopathic doctor, my approach to medicine is founded on these basic truths; whether I'm helping a patient tackle a disease like breast cancer or creating an ongoing preventative strategy so they can live a vibrant life.

The Basic Truths…

- The body's normal state is one of health and vibrancy.
- This normal state can be tipped off balance by an infinite number of factors both internal and external
- The body is **always** working to get back to its normal state.
- By correcting deficiencies and areas that are out of balance, the powerful and innate healing capacities are engaged and the body moves again toward health and vibrancy.

Being a naturopathic physician my goal is always to facilitate my patients return to extraordinary health. Guiding them to this state starts with a process of inquiry and investigation.

As you read this book, you are embarking on your own investigation. Inquiring how vitamin D can improve your health and that of your loved ones. This book will teach you to how to harness the powerful medicine in sunlight.

What's in store?

As you look inside these pages you will find:

- The startling statistics on your risk for acquiring diseases from vitamin D deficiency.
- How the sun gifts us with vitamin D and how our body brilliantly utilizes it to keep us healthy.
- How to reduce your risk of acquiring disease by maintaining optimal vitamin D levels.
- How cancer death rates can be drastically reduced by keeping healthy vitamin D levels in your blood.
- The latest research on safe dosages and a guide for optimal vitamin D levels.
- The determining factors that affect our daily supply of this vital nutrient.
- Other sources and forms of vitamin D if you don't get enough sunshine.
- How sunscreens not only inhibit our vitamin D skin production but can be potentially toxic, how to find safe sunscreens and how to effectively use them.
- How to safeguard your health and the health of your loved ones no matter where in the world you live or how much sunlight you're exposed to.
- Part II of this book is dedicated to preventing and healing from specific diseases and conditions related to vitamin D deficiency.

Natural medicine has already made huge advancements in preventing and/or shortening disease processes. It's my belief that established nutritional protocols along with the important adjunctive use of vitamin D therapy shall prove to be no less than true partners in health.

And finally, as a naturopathic physician, I can no longer dispute what I've intuitively believed in all along: the absence of sunshine creates a deficit of life supporting nutrients which keep us from attaining optimal health.

Chapter 2: The Unsettling Evidence

"Vitamin D is a hormone. Deficiencies of hormones can have catastrophic consequences."

Dr. William Davis, Cardiologist

For years now we've been scared out of the sun and, unfortunately, it has more to do with making money than reducing the risk of skin cancer and keeping us healthy. Sunscreen companies have been making billions of dollars by extolling the virtues of year round sunscreen use. They've even teamed up with the mega-rich cosmetic industry and successfully capitalized on our fear of wrinkles. These days it's commonplace to find facial products with added sunscreen and this is solely due to the demand they created.

Banning of the sun-worshippers

If you've been around a while, say since the 1970's or earlier, you likely remember a sun-worshipping era where hours in the sun and highly tanned skin were considered a competitive sport. But with big corporate funding from sunscreen and cosmetic companies to 'educate' the general public on dangers of skin cancer, this scene has dramatically changed. Our once overexposed, sun-loving society is now fearful. In fact, people who tan their skin are often scolded by their peers as being irresponsible. Parents are considered negligent if they let their children outside without sunscreen. And with all this strict sun-avoidance our culture is simultaneously experiencing dramatic rises in cancer, heart disease, auto-immune disease and decreases in mental health and our overall sense of well-being.

Farmers don't get cancer?

In 1941, the *Journal of Cancer* published a scientific study on farmers. An industry where people typically spend large amounts of time in the sun and where we get the phrase 'a farmers tan'. Oddly enough, scientists found that very few farmers developed cancers of the prostate, colon or breast. Their rates of acquiring these cancers were abnormally low compared to the general public. The scientists concluded that while these farmers showed increase in propensity to develop skin cancer, their time in the sun was providing an overall protective health benefit and preventing life threatening cancers.

Give me the numbers

To put the issue into perspective, 1,200 people die each year in the United States from non-melanoma skin cancer, a cancer attributed to overexposure to the sun. As a comparison, diseases which can be prevented by sun exposure and healthy vitamin D levels are killing hundreds of thousands of people every year in the United States. For example, colon and breast cancer, two cancers which are highly preventable with healthy levels of vitamin D, kill 138,000 individuals each year. By exposing our skin to the sun regularly and moderately these numbers would plummet.

In 1999, a definitive study by Dr. Ester John showed a direct link between breast cancer and vitamin D deficiency. After analyzing breast cancer statistics from the National Health and Nutrition Examination Survey, Dr. John stated that healthy blood levels of vitamin D -from sun exposure or supplementation in the diet- would significantly reduce the risk of developing and subsequently dying from breast cancer. In her study, a 35-75% decrease in diagnosis and death would occur through proper sun exposure.

In the United States alone, this means 100,000 new cases of breast cancer and 27,500 deaths each year could be prevented by sun exposure.

If those numbers seem unfathomable, it gets even better. With the combination of sun and supplementation with vitamin D, Dr. John estimated that the numbers of women spared this disease each year would increase to 150,000 and 37,500 respectively.

Breast cancer is just one cancer that can be prevented by keeping healthy blood levels of vitamin D. Prostate cancer kills 1 in 4 men diagnosed. In 2001, a study on prostate cancer was published in the prestigious scientific journal, The Lancet. Dr. Luscombe's study associated a lack of sun exposure to a decrease in the age at which men are diagnosed as well as an increase in overall susceptibility of developing the disease.

In another recent study at the University of California San Diego, Dr. Cedric Garland analyzed worldwide data on lung cancer. Statistics showed a marked increase in incidence of lung cancer as latitude increased. And an increase in latitude corresponds to a decrease in sunlight available for skin production of vitamin D.

Why is the time of year important?

In another study on lung cancer, the rate of survival after surgery directly correlated to the season. In the springtime, blood levels of vitamin D are typically at their lowest because of limited skin exposure to the sun in the wintertime. This is especially true at higher latitudes where the 'vitamin D winter' prevents vitamin D skin synthesis. Patients diagnosed with lung cancer in the springtime had a much higher rate of death after surgery then those diagnosed in the fall, when vitamin D levels are typically at their highest.

Death isn't the only consequence

Early death is not the only consequence of vitamin D deficiency. There are millions of people suffering and debilitated by conditions and diseases that can be prevented by and alleviated with vitamin D sufficiency.

In October of 2004 the Surgeon General issued a report on osteoporosis, a condition highly associated with vitamin D deficiency. The first thing mentioned on the fact sheet was that "weak bones should not be excused as a natural part of aging." It's estimated that in America, 10 million people suffer from osteoporosis. However, as many as 4 times that number of men and 3 times the number of women are actually affected by the disease and don't know it. Osteoporosis is considered the silent thief; because most people aren't diagnosed with osteoporosis until they fall and break a bone.

Each year 1.5 million Americans suffer bone fractures. The most common bone fractures happen to the wrist, spine and hip. It's estimated that 30% of people over 65 will experience a fall and consequent fracture. On average 13,700 people die each year from falls. The Surgeon General tells us that "hip fractures are the most devastating – 20% of people affected die within a year; 20% end up in nursing homes within a year; many become isolated and afraid to leave home because of fear of falling."

The link between sunlight (vitamin D) and improving bone health has been documented since the 1800's when Boston's Floating Hospital began taking children affected with the bone deforming rickets out on the water to get them into the sun. Yet today, the number of people affected by bone disease like osteoporosis, osteopenia and osteomalacia are dramatically rising. The surgeon general's report also gave us a warning, stating, "If immediate action is not taken, half of Americans over 50 will have weak bones from osteoporosis and low bone mass by 2020."

Vitamin D deficiency is tragically affecting children as well. Vitamin D experts Drs. Cannell and Hollis have recently published a study for physicians on the clinical use of vitamin D. In this study they have brought to light the convergence of epidemic cases of childhood autism, asthma and diabetes and the recommendation over the past few decades to slather sunscreen on children. The researchers noticed that the growing number of children affected with these diseases have, "blossomed after sun-avoidance advice became widespread..."

What can you do?

With all these frightening statistics on vitamin D deficiency and their link to disease, there is good news. By increasing blood levels of vitamin D you will engage an innate healing mechanism that your body can utilize to prevent and fight disease.

Chapter 3: The Politics of Sunshine

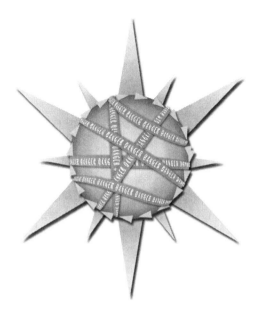

"Sunlight is more powerful than any drug; it is safe, effective, and available free of charge. If it could be patented, it would be hyped as the greatest medical breakthrough in history. It's that good."

<u>Mike Adams, Consumer Health Advocate</u>

So why don't more people know about the miraculous health benefits of vitamin D? With over 40 years of solid scientific evidence, why hasn't any changes to vitamin D dosing and RDA recommendations been urged to the public? Can we really blame politics and red tape? Unfortunately for our health, it's complicated...

Birth of the RDA

The RDA is the Recommended Daily Allowance of a number of different vitamins and minerals and is updated approximately every 10 years by the Institute of Medicine (IoM). The RDA was first designed as dietary recommendations for military personnel during World War II. After the war, it was decided that RDA's should be extrapolated to address the health needs of the entire nation. The transfer of responsibility for determining

RDA's moved from the military to the Institute of Medicine (IoM) and the National Academy of Sciences. Currently, the Food and Nutrition Board (FNB) at the Institute of Medicine is responsible for setting RDA's.

What is the purpose of the RDA?

Having an RDA seems like a great plan, except that the intention of the RDA has always been, and remains so today, to be the smallest quantity of a vitamin or mineral that will prevent most people from becoming seriously ill with debilitating deficiency diseases like scurvy (vitamin C), rickets (vitamin D) and beriberi (vitamin B1).

How is an RDA determined?

Before determining an RDA, the Food and Nutrition Board (FNB) needs to establish an EAR, which is an **E**stimated **A**verage **R**equirement. The FNB committee members first decide what criterion it wants to use to determine the EAR. For instance, they may decide to use research that conducted blood analysis or urine analysis. The IoM (Institute of Medicine) then selects from the hundreds of solid peer reviewed research articles, only those that meet their criteria. They then take this dwindled down pool of data and decide if an Estimated Average Requirement (EAR) can be determined.

If an EAR can be determined it means that at least 50% of the people in the study had their nutritional needs met. They then presume that this will apply to the entire population and they establish a bell-curve distribution and apply statistical data to determine the RDA. If an EAR cannot be established, an **A**dequate **I**ntake Level (AI) is determined, which is also an estimate based on their small pool of scientific data.

What if they don't have enough data?

The FNB faces another problem. Specifically, what to do when they do not have enough data about a particular gender or age group to make a determination. As you may already know, vitamin intake requirements change depending on gender, age, an increase or decrease in your activity level and if you are pregnant. The way the IoM has tackled this problem is to take information on another vitamin or mineral that has the data for that particular age or gender and they extrapolate the missing information and assume that it reacts similarly. As you may suspect, it could be dangerous work to make such assumptions. But, as long as the IoM keeps the RDA levels extremely low, they don't have to worry about recommending levels that are too high.

What does the IoM have to say?

When the IoM was questioned, Paula Trumbo, the Senior Program Officer of IoM's Food and Nutrition Board said, "Some of the RDA's are based on smaller samples. However, research indicates that for the most part, human metabolism varies within a fairly narrow range – so that 97% of the population falls within 20% of the bell-curve distribution. Most vitamins are enzyme cofactors, so the body's use of them is closely tied to metabolism."

Vitamin D doesn't fit in the IoM's mold

Unfortunately, when it comes to vitamin D it is not an enzyme cofactor and is not tied to metabolism. Vitamin D in its active form is regulated by the endocrine system and by specific tissues. The active form of vitamin D isn't a vitamin at all, it's a hormone.

Whose side of the fence are you on?

Another problem at the Institute of Medicine (IoM) is that the people who make up the committee are all coming at this from the same perspective. Dr. Jonathan Wright, a well known alternative health practitioner and author stated, "They are all coming from the same side of the fence. No one is looking at what might be called the natural medicine point of view." It's unfortunate for the health of the nation, that the organization charged with determining our vitamin intake does not have even one perspective or expert advisement from physicians trained in supporting the body with vitamins and minerals.

When it comes to vitamin D, we have an unsettling example of how the IoM functions. A few years ago an article was published in the American Journal of Clinical Nutrition, a peer reviewed research journal regarded as the leading publication in the field. Researchers in this field understand that the current 400 IU/day (for the 51-70 year age bracket) has only a modest effect on blood concentrations of vitamin D. Safety is the first priority when recommending advice on supplementation or fortification of any nutrient. With this in mind, researchers applied the risk assessment method used by the Food and Nutritional Board to update the safe tolerable upper limit (UL) for vitamin D. The conclusion was that the upper limit for vitamin D consumption by adults should be 10,000 IU/day. This indicates that the margin of safety for vitamin D consumption for adults is greater than 10 times any current recommended intake!!!

What research did the Institute of Medicine use to determine vitamin D's RDA?

Interestingly, the Institute of Medicine didn't use research on blood serum levels of vitamin D to determine its safe upper level. Instead it used serum calcium levels to make its determination. As you will see in Chapter 4: A Cellular Explanation, calcium levels are indeed related to vitamin D levels, but vitamin D also acts outside its relationship to calcium within specific tissues. So, why not use the plethora of data and research on serum levels of vitamin D? True to form for the Institute of Medicine, even the calcium serum level research they used for evaluating the safe upper levels were significantly higher than what they decided to recommend. Once again, giving us an extremely conservative recommendation where the actual research shows health benefits at much higher doses.

In the early 1970's, vitamin D serum concentrations thought to be 'adequate' were based simply on preventing rickets and osteomalacia. Yet, in 1997, some twenty years and hundreds of research article later, the IoM claimed they didn't have enough information to establish an EAR (Estimated Average Requirement) for vitamin D, and therefore could not define a RDA. An Adequate Intake (AI) was determined, which is the amount needed to maintain a defined nutritional state or criterion of adequacy, that is, the prevention of rickets or osteomalacia in the general population.

What is the current AI for vitamin D?

The current recommendations to the public by the Food and Nutrition Board for an adequate intake:

Age	IU's (Units)
Birth – 13	200 IU
14-18	200 IU
19-50	200 IU
Pregnancy	200 IU
Lactation	200 IU
51-70	400 IU
71 +	600 IU

Given that research has shown us that healthy individuals use upwards of 5,000 units everyday of vitamin D, and those combating illnesses use even more, these levels are drastically insufficient to maintain a healthy population. The FNB goes on to say that, "*The Adequate Intake level for vitamin D is based on the assumption that the vitamin is not synthesized by exposure to sunlight* ". This would be fine if they stressed the importance of getting additional vitamin D from the sun, however, they don't. In the Dietary Supplement Fact Sheet: Vitamin D, by the Office of Dietary Supplements at the National Institute of Health, it states, "Despite the importance of the sun to vitamin D synthesis, it is prudent to limit exposure of skin to sunlight." It goes on to say, "The American Academy of Dermatology advises that photoprotective measures be taken, including the use of sunscreen, whenever one is exposed to the sun."

Hmm, advising us to take minimal amounts of vitamin D and avoid the sun at all costs, surely doesn't sound like they have the health of the nation in mind!

What about the food industry?

The food industry has a vested interest in keeping RDA's low. For example, if the RDA (or AI) for vitamin D is 200 IU, a food packager can add 200 IU/serving to its milk and make the claim on the front of the package, *Get 100% of your RDA Vitamin D in every serving!* If the Food and Nutrition Board raised the RDA to a level that actually had a good protective benefit, such as 2,000 IU, the food packager would have to change their claim to, "*100% of your RDA in every 10 glasses*". Then we'd probably be inundated with advertisements on the importance of drinking 10 glasses of milk, daily.

In all seriousness, if the RDA was raised to sufficient levels, food packagers wanting to keep their claims would have to fortify their foods with a higher quantity of vitamins, which directly affects their bottom line.

What about the 800 lb. Gorilla?

Yet, I'm sure the Food and Nutrition Board at the Institute of Medicine and the food industry aren't the only reason that we don't know about the powerful medicinal effects of vitamin D. And when it comes to the words like *powerful* and *medicine*, one is inclined to think of an 800 pound gorilla known as the pharmaceutical industry. Obviously, Big Pharma's life line is through the sale drugs, and with a healthier population they would take a big hit to their bottom line. Especially since they can't package sunshine and sell it to us...or can they?

Big Pharma is very aware of how powerfully talented vitamin D really is. Since vitamin D can presumably prevent and cure hundreds of maladies

the drug, companies have been in a frenzy trying to come up with analogues (synthetic prototypes) of vitamin D, and sell them for profit. Some
research suggests that these analogues are not biocompatible with our
own tissues even though they may stimulate the Vitamin D Receptor sites
(VDR). And as with any synthetic analogue there is always a price to pay:
side effects.

Vitamin D is a natural vitamin and cannot be patented and thus 'sold' by
the pharmaceutical companies. From Big Pharma's point of view, there is
little or no interest in pursuing public education/marketing. If the industry actually promoted the analogue via a mass media campaign the same
way they do their other drugs, this would cause people to start asking
questions, like: *"Is vitamin D anti-carcinogenic? If I get out in the sun will
I be healthier?"* If you, the public, learned how critically important vitamin
D was to your health, you would likely make changes that would leave you
healthier and less likely to need the drugs the pharmaceutical companies
are so desperately trying to push.

A circular information trap

Part of it is a system problem...a circular information trap. It works something like this...a researcher at a University wants to conduct research on
vitamin D. To conduct the research the professor needs to have funding
so they apply for a grant from the National Institute of Health (NIH). The
NIH is a government funded institution and one of the things it does is to
provide grants to companies and universities. These monies are dispersed
to qualified projects and preference is given to research in which they are
specifically interested. For instance, if the Institute of Medicine has determined it needs more research in a particular area for RDA recommendations, preference and funding will be given for that research.

The NIH does this through a Program Announcement (PA) and a Request
for Application (RFA). The Program Announcement "identifies areas of
increased priority and/or emphasis for a specific area of science. More
specifically, the RFA identifies a more narrowly defined area for which one
or more NIH institutes have set aside funds for awarding grants."
(http://grants.nih.gov/grants/guide/description.htm)

How are the Universities funded?

You may have assumed that Universities are funded by the government
and the tuition students pay to attend. This is only partly true. A vast

amount of the money comes from research grants. This is why many pro-fessors are not only encouraged to do research in addition to teaching, they are required to. A professor who wants to keep the grants flowing will submit grant proposals with research designed to obtain funds that have been pre-allocated by the NIH. In this way, the government is con-trolling the "independent" research conducted at the Universities.

Another source of income for the Universities is from corporations need-ing independent product research. Corporations that submit information to the FDA and EPA for approval and claims are required to have inde-pendent evaluations. This seems to be good for everyone; the University is financially compensated, the corporation gets a professional evaluation, and the professor can use the research to publish a paper on the subject if they choose to. Being published in prestigious journals as a professor is important for their career. It's also good to note that research funded by private companies is most often designed by those companies with the desire for obtaining specific information.

What happens to the research?

After a grant is awarded and research conducted, a research paper detail-ing the findings is submitted to peer reviewed journals for possible pub-lishing. If the paper is selected, the journal sets a date and chooses when it would be appropriate for this article to be published. From inception to completion this process takes years.

After the journal is published, it is read by other peers interested in simi-lar research. And, as so often is the case, the results from research serve to identify areas where further research is needed. A few different things happen at this point. First, nothing may come of it. Second, another researcher, or perhaps the same one may apply for another grant to answer the questions raised in the latest research. Or third, an interested researcher may do a complete review of all the literature on the subject and publish an article summarizing what we know so far and again identi-fying areas where further research is needed.

Is the process becoming clear? It's a system of applying for grants, conduct-ing research, publishing, determining further research needed, applying for another grant, doing more research, and so on. This system is vitally important and one that is always aspiring to learn and understand more.

A frustrated scientific community

In the case of vitamin D, a knowledge gap exists where important and relevant information generated by research, directly applicable to improving health, is not being provided to the public – either not at all, or at least not in a responsible way. The researchers who've diligently research year after year and published article after article praising vitamin D and purporting its vital role in the human body, are extremely frustrated over the same old vitamin D information being reported by the media.

For over 40 years, the scientific community has reported in a vast array of medical journals, including the prestigious American Journal of Clinical Nutrition and the Journal of the American Medical Association, pointing out the significant health effects and widespread deficiency of vitamin D, yet no real changes have being made. It's no wonder why these researchers are frustrated; the IoM and the media continue to obscure the published evidence, leaving it 'stuck' in the circular information trap of publications that continues documenting the same old vitamin D inadequacy. As long as this continues, people will continue getting sick and dying of diseases that could otherwise be prevented.

The vitamin D researcher's modus operandi is to protect and improve the health of the public. They know the realities of serum vitamin D concentrations around the globe. The have concluded that public health would dramatically benefit from improved 'D' nutritional status. They know the intakes of vitamin D needed to help improve the public's health. So why is it that the scientific evidence has not made any impact on public health?

Those most familiar with the research, other than the researchers themselves, are the government, media, and companies with a vested interest. Unfortunately, the information in the research doesn't even come close to matching the information provided to us by our trusted institutions or the media. Something is a miss.

A lack of pressure on policy makers – a misleading media

The scientific community believes the reason no appreciable changes have been made is due to the lack of pressure on policy makers. Public pressure always carries a lot of weight; however, misinformation from outdated sources still gets propagated by the media. This could stem from a concern over possible litigation if the media were to advise a 'toxic' intake greater than or equal to the current upper limit. The media often reports to us in a manner leaving us believing we don't need to take action. You may read something like this; *"Current recommendations from the Institute of Medicine call for 200 IU/day from birth through age 50, 400 IU/day for ages 51-70, and 600 IU/day for those older than 70 years. Some experts say that optimal amounts are closer to 1,000 IU daily. Until more is known it is not safe to overdo it,"* and conclude that it may be dangerous to go over the RDA. This misinformation results in little public pressure and minimal motivation for policy makers to implement the relatively simple steps needed to correct this deficiency.

The consequences of a drastically low RDA

The serious health consequences on our society caused by governmental guidance to recommend the smallest amount that will prevent serious diseases can be seen everywhere. Our bodies are deficient in vitamin D. Rickets, the bone deforming disease affecting children, once thought to be completely cured, is now on the rise. And what are the long term effects of vitamin D deficiency? In the United States alone, 10 million people, men and women, are afflicted with osteoporosis and another 30 million are affected by osteopenia (a less severe bone loss disease). And let's not forget the drastic rise in cancers of the breast, ovaries, prostate and lungs and people affected with non-specific pain disorder, depression, seasonal affected disorder (SAD) and MS.

What the public needs -

Ultraviolet B light is an overwhelmingly greater source of vitamin D than is food or supplements. And research tells us that the recommended daily allowance needs to be a much higher daily dose! The National correction of low vitamin D status in our population will only happen if the public is urged to make changes such as encouragement of optimal doses of sun exposure, eating 'D' fortified foods and increasing vitamin D supplementation to a truly adequate level.

Overall, these are all low budget changes. If implemented they may very well bring about rapid and severe reductions in the morbidity associated with low vitamin D levels.

It's up to you

Yes indeed, if Big Pharma can't stuff its pockets with profits, they will be of no use in helping the public recognize the miraculous benefits of vitamin D. It is unlikely the government and big corporations are going to help with widespread education of vitamin D. It's up to you, the public to make a difference.

So, take the bull by its horns and become proactive in your own healthcare! Read the research, have your physician evaluate an optimal dose of vitamin D for you and have your serum levels checked regularly.

Meanwhile, as public supporters of vitamin D, we urge you to change public healthcare policies by putting pressure on the media, vitamin manufacturers and congressmen to undertake new initiatives that will have a realistic chance of making a difference in vitamin D health. Obviously, there's a major need to internationally re-access vitamin D dietary recommendations and change outdated policies and recommendations.

Chapter 4: A Cellular Explanation

"Humans make thousands of units of vitamin D within minutes of whole body exposure to sunlight. From what we know of nature, it is unlikely such a system evolved by chance."

Dr. Cannell, Executive Director, Vitamin D Council
www.vitamindcouncil.org

To thoroughly grasp vitamin D's powerful impact in our body, it's essential to take a look inside and to see exactly how it functions. The branch of biology devoted to these internal activities is called physiology. Human physiology is the study of vital and essential processes that our bodies naturally undertake to maintain life.

A heart and lungs example

We all know that the heart is critical for life and the basic function of the heart is simply to keep blood circulating throughout our body. This circulating blood contains vital nutrients that are delivered to the body. Oxygen is just one of those nutrients and the physiology goes like this:

a. The heart pumps de-oxygenated blood to the lungs, then
b. the lungs transfer oxygen to the blood, then
c. the heart pumps the oxygenated blood back to the heart, then
d. the heart pumps this blood to the body through the arteries, then
e. the tissues of our body pull the oxygen out of the blood and transfer it to the cells to be used to fuel the vital processes inside the cells, then
f. the de-oxygenated blood returns to the heart via the veins to be re-oxygenated by the lungs, and the cycle begins again.

For this process to function optimally, our lungs need to be in good shape, the heart needs to be strong to continuously pump blood to the lungs and the body, the blood needs to contain iron which binds the oxygen and delivers it to the tissues and our arteries and veins need to be clear to allow the fluids to pass freely. When even one system is not functioning optimally we notice. If our iron is low, we're tired; if our lungs are infected we find ourselves coughing, tired and short of breath.

What's the point?

The point is this: our physiology is tightly regulated by the body, so that when we are out of balance, symptoms begin to show up. Symptoms are our body's way of telling us something is out of whack. With the help of a knowledgeable physician they can find out what is going on and take steps to move us back to equilibrium.

Houston, we have a problem

However, when it comes to vitamin D deficiency we've had a problem. Until recently, most doctors didn't understand the powerful role vitamin D plays in preventing and curing disease. If you were diagnosed with cancer, your vitamin D levels would not be checked and supplementation would not be considered as part of a treatment plan. With the persistence of researchers in this field, this scenario is now changing.

So how does the vitamin D work in our body? As humans we can obtain vitamin D from three different sources; first, by exposing our skin to UVB rays in sunlight (or from a tanning bed); second, by taking nutritional supplementation or prescribed vitamin D; and third, through eating foods naturally containing vitamin D and those that are fortified.

The most effective and abundant source of vitamin D comes in the form of sunlight. Now while there are many variables that affect our ability to utilize sunlight for vitamin D production, for now let's assume it's a clear sunny day, we live in an area with relatively low air pollution and little ozone interference allowing the sunrays to reach the earth's surface, and we are in one of the southern states in the US, or it's summertime elsewhere. Assuming these factors are in place, then sunlight can work its magic in our skin.

How does the magic work?

Our skin has a variety of cells. Two competing cells are those with melanin pigmentation and cells with a molecule called 7-dehydroxycholesterol (7DHC). Melanin is the pigmentation that gives skin its color. The more cells you have with active melanocytes the fewer you have with 7DHC, and the darker your skin. Conversely, the fewer cells with active melanocytes the more with 7DHC and the lighter your skin. Melanin helps protect against sunburn, skin damage and skin cancer and people with darker skin can tolerate much longer amounts of time in the sun. It's nature's sunblock.

So, we're outside on a sunny day and a photon of sunlight reaches a skin cell containing 7DHC. This skin cell is then photoisomerized into previtamin D_3. (Photoisomerisation is a fancy name to describe using sunlight to change the form of 7DHC into previtamin D3.) The photons of sunlight that accomplish this task are shorter than 315nm in wavelength which makes the UVB spectrum (290-315nm) the only wavelengths that our skin can utilize to make previtamin D_3. Now, for the next several hours, a heat isomerisation in the skin *slowly* converts the previtamin D_3 to vitamin D_3.

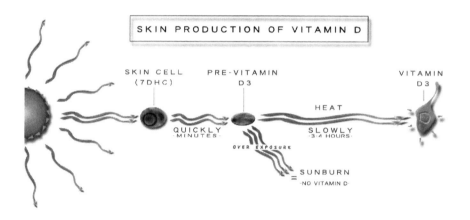

If you're thinking more time in the sun is better...think again.

Lots of time in the sun ≠ more vitamin D_3 ≠ healthier

By exposing skin longer than necessary to make previtamin D_3 another process kicks in whereby the previtamin D_3 is further photoconverted to either lumisterol or tachysterol (two inert isomers) or back to 7DHC. It is therefore, not only unnecessary and unneeded to spend lots of time in the sun with unprotected skin and risking sunburn, but it actually decreases the available previtamin D_3 to be converted to vitamin D_3 that could have been utilized by the body.

Once vitamin D_3 is made in the skin it is picked up by a vitamin D-binding protein (DBP) and enters the blood stream where it is taken to the liver to be metabolized into 25-hydroxyvitamin D, or **25(OH)D** as it is referred to by vitamin D experts and your physician.

Blood levels of 25(OH)D are measured by your physician to accurately determine your vitamin D health. 25(OH)D is not the active form of vitamin D that is actually used, but rather the form that is available for the kidneys, tissues and organs to pull off the shelf and convert as needed.

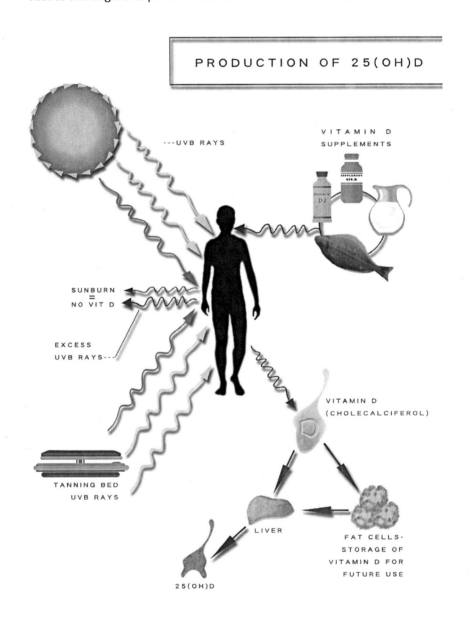

PRODUCTION OF 25(OH)D

---UVB RAYS

VITAMIN D
SUPPLEMENTS

SUNBURN
=
NO VIT D

EXCESS
UVB RAYS---

TANNING BED
UVB RAYS

VITAMIN D
(CHOLECALCIFEROL)

LIVER

FAT CELLS-
STORAGE OF
VITAMIN D FOR
FUTURE USE

25(OH)D

Not all vitamin D is created equally

Now here is where vitamin D from supplements, food sources and fortified foods come in to play. Vitamin D_3 (calciferol) is found in natural food sources, some fortified foods and most over the counter vitamins. Vitamin D_2 (ergocalciferol) is the form found in some fortified foods as well as prescribed vitamin D. Both forms bind equally well to the vitamin D-binding protein and are carried to the liver for processing. The liver metabolizes D_2 and D_3 to $25(OH)D_2$ and $25(OH)D_3$, respectively.

Vitamin D_2 was once thought to be on equal standing in effectiveness as vitamin D_3 as both provide a relatively equal rise in serum $25(OH)D$ levels. However, once metabolized in the liver, a sharp divergence occurs as the serum $25(OH)D_2$ rapidly declines over a few days whereas serum $25(OH)D_3$ rises and maintains a higher blood level for a significantly longer period of time. Dr. Armas, published research showing vitamin D_3's superior efficacy is up to 10-fold greater than vitamin D_2 - a fact which must be considered by your physician, when recommending effective dosing.

Making of the ACTIVE FORM

So, now we have a circulating serum level of $25(OH)D$ that physicians can measure and determine if a deficiency exists. This circulating form is the best indicator of vitamin D status, but it is not the active form that imparts miraculous health benefits. No, we now need to travel to the kidneys to further metabolize it into 1,25-dihydroxyvitamin D, or $1,25(OH)_2D$ – the active form!

At this point, the active form is considered a hormone as it becomes part of a complex endocrine biofeedback system. The levels of active vitamin D hormone are self-limiting and tightly regulated by calcium and phosphorus levels and the parathyroid hormone (PTH). If the levels become too low, the parathyroid hormone (PTH) increases which stimulate the kidneys to convert the circulating serum levels of $25(OH)D$ into 1-$25(OH)_2D$. If the levels become too high, the parathyroid hormone levels decrease which in turn decrease the synthesis of $1,25(OH)_2D$ in the kidneys. Excessive levels of $1,25(OH)_2D$ are broken down by the same enzyme used for synthesizing it into the inactive calcitroic acid. The programming of its own destruction (activated vitamin D) is an important hallmark of the endocrine system.

This is where the powerful medicine happens

The activated form of vitamin D is considered to be the most powerful pleiotropic hormone that is produced in our bodies, acting on over 200 genes. The powerful effects begin when an activated vitamin D binds to a vitamin D receptor (VDR). This complex has a myriad of affects on the body.

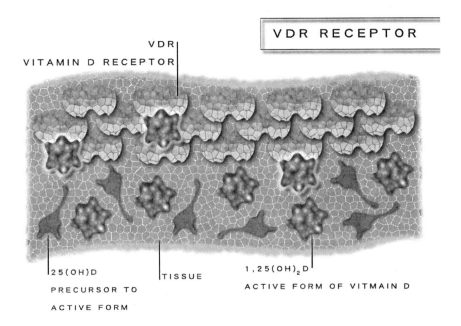

VDR
VITAMIN D RECEPTOR

VDR RECEPTOR

25(OH)D
PRECURSOR TO
ACTIVE FORM

TISSUE

1,25(OH)$_2$D
ACTIVE FORM OF VITMAIN D

The amazing discovery!

It has long been held that the kidneys were the only place that converts serum vitamin D into its active form. What has proved to be true, however, is that specific tissues in the body have their own independent activation factories. When there is not enough activated vitamin D produced by the kidneys, a 'back up' kicks in wherein the tissues themselves are able to take circulating 25(OH)D out of the blood and convert it to its active form. This is absolutely amazing!

From an evolutionary perspective, this 'back up' system exists to protect the body and keep it healthy. It may also represent the increased demand these particular tissues have for vitamin D as their importance in the proper functioning of the body cannot be understated. What we also know is that whenever a tissue is combating an illness, like an auto-immune disease or cancer, the tissue requirements for vitamin D are significantly higher.

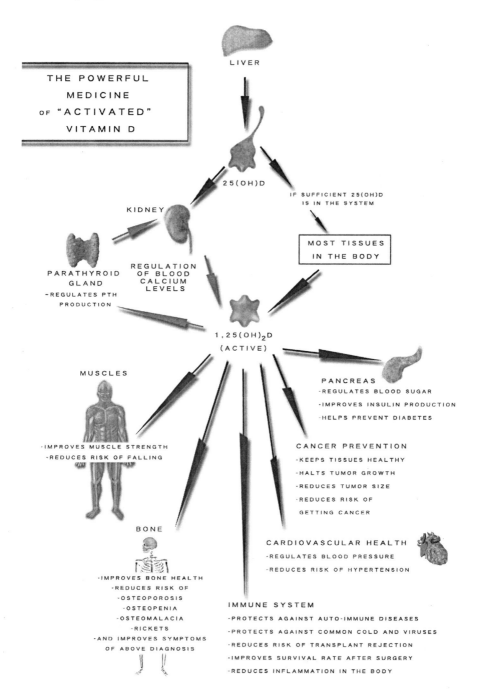

THE POWERFUL MEDICINE OF "ACTIVATED" VITAMIN D

LIVER

25(OH)D

KIDNEY

IF SUFFICIENT 25(OH)D IS IN THE SYSTEM

MOST TISSUES IN THE BODY

PARATHYROID GLAND
-REGULATES PTH PRODUCTION

REGULATION OF BLOOD CALCIUM LEVELS

1,25(OH)$_2$D (ACTIVE)

MUSCLES

PANCREAS
-REGULATES BLOOD SUGAR
-IMPROVES INSULIN PRODUCTION
-HELPS PREVENT DIABETES

-IMPROVES MUSCLE STRENGTH
-REDUCES RISK OF FALLING

CANCER PREVENTION
-KEEPS TISSUES HEALTHY
-HALTS TUMOR GROWTH
-REDUCES TUMOR SIZE
-REDUCES RISK OF GETTING CANCER

BONE

CARDIOVASCULAR HEALTH
-REGULATES BLOOD PRESSURE
-REDUCES RISK OF HYPERTENSION

-IMPROVES BONE HEALTH
-REDUCES RISK OF
-OSTEOPOROSIS
-OSTEOPENIA
-OSTEOMALACIA
-RICKETS
-AND IMPROVES SYMPTOMS OF ABOVE DIAGNOSIS

IMMUNE SYSTEM
-PROTECTS AGAINST AUTO-IMMUNE DISEASES
-PROTECTS AGAINST COMMON COLD AND VIRUSES
-REDUCES RISK OF TRANSPLANT REJECTION
-IMPROVES SURVIVAL RATE AFTER SURGERY
-REDUCES INFLAMMATION IN THE BODY

Examples of how optimal levels of active vitamin D functions in our body:

- Improved muscle performance. A positive relationship exists between optimal vitamin D serum levels and physical performance. This is because muscle cells carry large quantities of vitamin D receptors. Research has shown that when serum levels were above 60nmol (24ng/ml) the muscle function tests (walking/chair standing) showed optimal performance

- Reduced risk of falling and of fracture: Improved muscle performance means we have better balance which naturally protects us from falling. If a fall occurs, having optimal serum levels of vitamin D ensure normal bone mineralization and healthy bones which resist breakage or heal faster if they do break.

- Protection against osteoporosis, osteopenia and osteomalacia: Research has shown that the number of vitamin D receptors decreased with age. This explains our even greater need for vitamin D from the sun and/or as supplementation. As we age, we become at greater risk for osteoporosis, osteopeneia, autoimmune disorders and cancers.

- Protection against cancer. Years of research have shown a relationship between lower sunshine exposure and higher cancer prevalence and cancer mortality. By having optimal serum levels, genes are 'turned on' to promote cellular differentiation. This allows the body to tell the difference between a cancer cell to get rid of and a normal healthy cell to keep.

- Halting the growth of tumors and inducing their breakdown. At optimal vitamin D serum levels, genes are activated to stop the growth of, or suppress proliferation of cancer cells. Activated vitamin D metabolites 'turn off' inflammatory markers such as IL-2 and IL-12. These active metabolites thus have the 'ability' to control cancerous growths because of their anti-proliferation (anti-growth) effects, by down-regulating dedridic cells and T-helper cells. Suppression of the antigen presenting capacity of macrophages and promotion of Th2 lymphocytes is an important part of the anti-'autoimmune'process that vitamin D imparts.

- Vitamin D's direct role in the immune system: Studies have shown that a vitamin D deficiency helps to activate the immune system; especially T-cell mediated immunity. Whereas, vitamin D in high doses actually suppresses certain aspects of the immune system. Vitamin D's role in the immune system has been shown in its remarkable ability to affect multiple sclerosis, diabetes, lupus, fibromyalgia and non-specific pain disorder.

- Multiple Sclerosis: activated vitamin D has been shown to prevent autoimmune encephalomyelitis, the experimental (animal model) of multiple sclerosis. Scientists found that this disease could be suppressed or eliminated at any stage of development with adequate amounts of vitamin D hormone administered orally each day. Another study showed that a higher sun exposure at an age of 6-15 years was associated with a lower risk of MS.

- Lupus, irritable bowel and rheumatoid arthritis: Similar results to those found for multiple sclerosis, were obtained with models of systemic lupus, irritable bowel disease and rheumatoid arthritis.

- Suppression of diabetes mellitus. Vitamin D also positively affects pancreatic beta cells and improves insulin sensitivity. Among non-obese diabetic rates, vitamin D deficiency caused a marked increase in incidence and a substantial decrease in lag time required for the onset of diabetes. In fact, large doses of vitamin D hormone could suppress type I diabetes mellitus completely by preventing the destruction of islet cells.

- Suppression of transplant rejection. An extended example of the autoimmune suppressive quality of vitamin D is a study demonstrating how activated vitamin D helps prevent transplant rejection in both vascular and nonvascular transplants.

A likely scenario for the suppression of these autoimmune diseases involves the vitamin D hormone interacting with the T-helper lymphocytes, which in turn suppress the inflammatory responses of T-helper type 1 lymphocytes. Although the exact mechanism of this regulation of autoimmune diseases is not understood, the results are substantial enough to warrant further investigation of vitamin D and possibly a synthetic analogue.

What about analogues?

An analogue is a synthetic copycat of the real thing. Since vitamin D has clearly shown its natural abilities to help prevent a myriad of diseases; pharmaceutical companies have been in a frenzy to create the perfect analogue.

One reason synthetic analogues are actively being designed to mimic natural vitamin D is in fact due to its dose limiting effects. With the kidneys closely regulating the quantity of activated vitamin D, this can limit the amount available for tissues and organs. This is especially important for tissues without a "back-up" system to make there own activated form. An important design consideration when creating synthetic analogues is to eliminate vitamin D's calcium increasing activity. Most analogue development in this field has been done with this in mind. Although, it appears in other studies that part of the immune system regulation requires increased calcium serum levels.

There's nothing like the real thing, baby!

Even if a synthetic analogue were developed to mimic vitamin D's effects there is no comparison with what mother-nature has already created. The design of analogues to treat a disease other than osteoporosis must include the elimination of this plasma calcium increasing activity. While these new vitamin D designer drugs will be able to treat cancers and other diseases, they will be cost prohibitive for many, yet make millions for the pharmaceutical companies. Natural vitamin D is free from the sun and inexpensive to take as a daily supplement.

The classification debate: Is vitamin D a vitamin or a hormone?

Currently there is quite a bit of debate about whether vitamin D is actually a vitamin because it is not utilized 'as is' directly by the body, but must be bio-chemically processed before it becomes active.

Once processed and converted to its active form, vitamin D is recognized by the body as a hormone. In its active form vitamin D binds to the vitamin D receptor site (VDR). Binding to this site turns on the genetic controls for that particular tissue.

The prospect of having vitamin D reclassified as something other than a vitamin presents interesting consequences. Perhaps the governance of its dosage recommendations will fall away from the Institute of Medicine who only recommends the smallest amount possible to hopefully prevent serious disease.

As far as this book is concerned, whether vitamin D gets reclassified is not as important as addressing the widespread deficiencies that occur from its lack. For now, let's find a way to protect our health and reap the benefits of it, no matter what it's called.

Chapter 5: What's blocking your sun?

"Even light white cotton, plain weave cloth prevents vitamin D photosynthesis"

Dr. Matsuoka, et.al.
Clothing prevents Ultraviolet-B Radiation-Dependent photosynthesis of vitamin D3.

Our bodies NEED the sun...just like flowers need the rain.

You can see it now. Sunlight is an essential component for healthy living. With it we are happier and healthier, we can withstand winters without getting ill, our bodies can fend off cancers and our immune system functions optimally. Life is good!

But without it, when we become deficient in vitamin D, life looks a whole lot different. We may not be able to put our finger on it at first, but over time it takes on a number of disguises. Depression, muscle fatigue, mental fogginess, bone aches and pains, the list goes on. What is happening to our body? Why isn't it working as well as it used to? In this case, it isn't age that's getting to us, it's that our body is lacking the vitamin D resources to pull from to mount a fight. Unfortunately, a vitamin D deficiency over any prolonged period of time, ultimately results in illness, disease and even death.

I have become convinced intellectually of something I've intuitively known all along. We need the sun. We're ready for it. We've missed it and now we have permission to once again sit under her rays and let her warm our skin and heal our bodies.

Okay, so what's blocking your sun?

There are lots of things blocking you. Some are environmental, some are personal, and some are simply facts of life. But all of them, individually and cumulatively, affect how much sunlight you'll get and consequently how much vitamin D your skin makes.

At the end of this chapter you'll find a flow chart to help you determine how and when you can best get your vitamin D from sunlight, and when you can't. When free sunlight is unavailable or inconvenient, you'll need to explore other ways of supplementing.

The Environment

You're environment plays a major role in your sunlight consumption and the ability for your body to synthesize vitamin D. Everything from where you live to the amount of ozone in the air directly affects your vitamin D levels. Here are the variables:

What does my latitude have to do with it?

You're latitude is the distance you live north or south of the equator and is measured in degrees. It's important to know your latitude because it affects how much 'effective' sunlight you are exposed to throughout the year.

What do I mean by 'effective' sunlight? Well, you could be outside on a warm sunny day in February, but if you're living above 42 degrees latitude, no vitamin D will be synthesized in your skin. Why? Because of something called a SZA (solar zenith angle). During the wintertime, at higher latitudes, the sun's rays must travel a greater distance to reach the earth's surface. The higher the latitude the further it must travel. And the further it travels the less intense and effective it becomes. By the time it reaches the earth's surface the effective UVB rays are diminished to the point of being ineffective for vitamin D synthesis. The result is no vitamin D can be made in your skin during those winter months. In general, if your latitude is above 40 degrees north or south of the equator you will likely benefit from supplementing with other sources during your vitamin D winter.

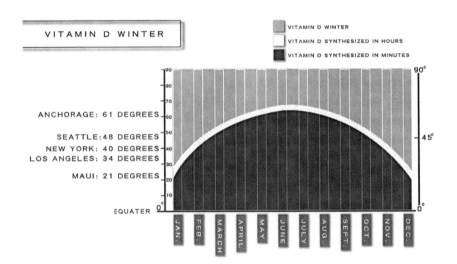

How big of a deal is our latitude really? Numerous studies have shown that people who live closer to the equator have a lower incidence of cancers, autoimmune diseases, hypertension, strokes, heart disease and depression.

The SZA: or where are you and what time is it?

Technically, the SZA (solar zenith angle) is the angle between the local vertical and the direct solar beam. A small SZA means the distance the UVB rays travel to the earth's surface is shorter, giving us more effective sunlight for vitamin D synthesis in the skin. Conversely, a long SZA means the sun's rays must travel further. By traveling a longer distance the sun's rays are dispersed and become less potent for vitamin D synthesis.

Small SZA's are associated with solar noon, summer and low latitudes. Long SZA's are associated with early morning/late evening, winter and higher latitudes.

Let's say you've determined your latitude and it's currently a season where you make vitamin D in your skin. The next consideration is the time of day you choose to spend in the sun. Based on the SZA's, if you want the most bang for your buck (most effective for the least amount of time) pick a time around your solar noon. Solar noon is the point where the sun is at its highest in the sky. This may vary considerably from twelve o'clock due to daylight savings time and your particular time zone.

I'm singing in the rain.

Rain is wonderful. For starters, it gives us our green trees, waters our gardens and fills our reservoirs. What it also does is block our sunlight. It doesn't even have to be raining either. It could just be threatening to rain by covering us with thick cloud cover. Those clouds directly filter out the UVB rays. We can tell it is daylight outdoors, but we won't be feeling the sun on our skin. If you live in an area like Seattle, where a good part of the year it will be cloudy, it's highly likely that you are deficient in vitamin D. Dense cloud cover and relatively few days every year with effective sunlight is enough to warrant supplementing with another source of vitamin D for a good part of the year.

I can't breathe...

Air pollutants and aerosols also reduce the amount of UVB rays reaching the earth's surface. They do this by scattering and absorbing sunlight. One of the signs of air pollution is a clogged up nose. Obviously, there are lots of other causes of nasal congestion and drainage such as allergies and the common cold. However, if you live in an area with lots of air pollution you may be suffering from nasal and sinus congestion as well as vitamin D deficiency. By the way, clogging your nose and sinuses is your body's way of protecting you from pollutants.

Ozone...Ozone...Ozone

Ozone is one of the major absorbers of UVB radiation. Ozone is located in our stratosphere and is always moving. There is however, some predictability to ozone distribution and thickness. Ozone is at its minimum near the equator and it increases in density as it moves further north and south. This is important to note because latitude is one of the major factors affecting vitamin D levels. Numerous studies have shown us that the further north or south of the equator we go, the more overall vitamin D levels decrease.

Reflectivity

There are also surface variances that increase UVB rays coming through the atmosphere. UVB rays increase when they encounter reflective surfaces such as water and fresh snow. The effect of these reflective surfaces increases again when cloud cover is present. When UVB rays reach a reflective surface they bounce back toward the atmosphere and we are thereby exposed twice to the same rays (once on the way down and once on bounce back). If a cloud is present the rays bounce off the clouds and again back down to us. In this way we are being exposed over and over to the same UVB rays. Under a high concentration of UVB our potential for getting sunburned increases dramatically. This is why it's easier to get sunburned when you're on the water or when you're snow skiing.

What do I have to do with it?

The environment determines whether or not UVB is available to us. But once that is established, it's the personal factors that individually affect the amount of vitamin D we are able to produce.

Age – one of the facts of life…

As we age so does our skin. There have been many studies demonstrating reduced levels of vitamin D in elderly people. There are several reasons for this such as: poor diet, lack of sun exposure and poor oral supplementation. Most elderly people don't spend much time in the sun. Their days of sitting outside on the front porch have been dwindling as they're placed in nursing homes where they rarely get enough natural sunlight.

If you are confined to a nursing home you are probably extremely deficient in vitamin D. One highly respected researcher suggests oral dosing all nursing home residents at 50,000 IU once a month.

Dietary influences also play a big role. Although diet is not the most effective way to raise vitamin D levels, because it is not naturally occurring in most foods, there are some that are fortified. (See Chapter 5: Finding your optimal dose for a list of foods containing vitamin D). As we age, food choices become poor, mostly due to convenience and cost.

Another important factor which further reduces our vitamin D levels is that as our skin ages, we have fewer cells containing 7DHC (the cells in the epidermis which produce pre-vitamin D). As a result, our ability to convert sunlight into vitamin D is reduced.

Science has shown that our skin cells capacity for making vitamin D begins to slow down after the age of 49. In addition, other studies have linked increased bone loss after age 49 to deficient vitamin D levels. In part, this is a result of declining hormone levels, sedentary lifestyles and poor diet. Overall, as our skin's capacity to make vitamin D decreases as we age, we begin to see the affects of its deficiency everywhere.

What about the babies?

On the other end of this age continuum are babies. Babies have also been found to be very deficient in vitamin D. This has manifested in a rise in the bone-deforming rickets, as wells as increased incidence of asthma, autism and diabetes in children.

While breastfeeding is a great way to provide the 'perfect food' for your baby, breast milk often does not supply your baby with adequate quantities of vitamin D, because the mother is often times vitamin D deficient herself. Studies have shown that vitamin D deficient mothers only produced 15-40 IU of vitamin D in their breast milk. Because vitamin D is important in the developing brain, it's important to supplement.

> **"As most breast milk contains little or no vitamin D, breast-fed babies should take 1,000 IU per day as a supplement unless they are exposed to sunlight. The only exception to this are lactating mothers who either get enough sun exposure or take enough vitamin D (usually 4,000–6,000 IU per day) to produce breast milk that is rich in vitamin D." Dr. Cannell; Vitamin D Expert, www.vitamindcouncil.org**

If a baby is fed formula, the formula is likely fortified with vitamin D2, in which case, absorption can be an issue. Dr. Cannell, recommends formula fed babies to take an extra 600 IU per day until they are weaned and then take 1,000 IU a day, until they are over 1.

Another age particularly at risk for deficiency is the 12 to 18 month old child. It's at this age when toddlers are often weaned from formula and or the breast. When this happens, and if they are not exposed to regular sunlight, their vitamin D levels drop. Vitamin D supplementation for children is recommended whenever regular sun exposure is limited.

Now you're telling me that skin color does matter?

It does when it comes to determining how much time to spend in the sun to synthesize vitamin D. In fact, skin color is a major consideration.

Melanin is the pigment in our skin that gives it color. Melanin is produced by melanocytes in our skins top layer, the epidermis. Everyone has relatively equal numbers of melanocytes in their skin. The difference in skin color arises because of the activity within these cells. People with lighter skin have a regularly low activity level within the melanocyte, whereas people with the darkest skin have highly active melanocytes.

Skin color is established by the regular activity level within the melanocyte. In addition to this regular activity, melanocytes can be induced into action by exposure to the sun. Our experience of 'getting a tan' is the result of that process.

Nature's sunblock

Melanin is our body's way of producing sun-block. More melanin in our skin means stronger protection and more time spent outdoors without burning. What this natural sun-block also does is slow down skin cell production of vitamin D by absorbing UVB rays.

As a result, the darker your skin, the more time you can spend in the sun without burning *and* the more time you'll need to stay in the sun to make vitamin D. For lighter skin this means you produce vitamin D in your skin faster, but you cannot stay in the sun as long without damaging your skin.

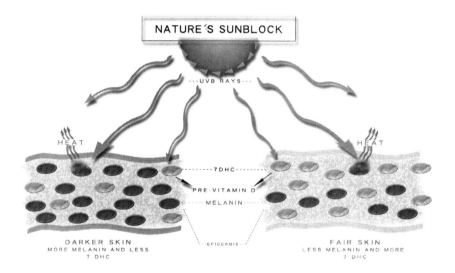

The lightest skin types are type 1 and 2 and typically require about 30 minutes or less in the sun to make the maximum dose of vitamin D. Type 3 and 4 skin types require approximately three times that amount or an hour and half. The darkest skin types, 5 and 6 may actually need up to 3 hours in the sun to obtain the desired affect. These estimates are for optimal sunlight (solar noon). The later or earlier in the day it is, the longer you will need to be in the sun to get the same effect.

As you consider your own time requirements as well as your lifestyle, you may find it necessary to supplement with vitamin D as long periods of time in the sun aren't attainable for most of us, especially if we work indoors.

Ideally, with each skin type, when you are in the sun, you'll want have your skin unprotected from the sun's rays only long enough to get your daily dose of vitamin D. After that, please cover up or use sunscreen to protect your skin.

If you recall from Chapter 4: A Cellular Explanation, longer periods of time in the sun do not equate to more vitamin D. Once pre-vitamin D is made in the skin, the skin becomes saturated and needs the next few hours to process it into vitamin D. By keeping your skin uncovered longer than necessary you are not only risking sunburn and potentially skin cancer, but are initiating another process that actually breaks down pre-vitamin D - making it useless for our bodies.

For more information on melanin, skin type and sunlight requirements please refer to Chapter 7: Shedding Light on Skin Cancer and Skin Health.

What about my health?

In Chapter 6: Finding your optimal dose, you'll find a list of the types of drugs that interfere with vitamin D synthesis as well as implicated health conditions which require special attention.

What about my weight?

Weight is an important variable in the process of raising vitamin D levels and keeping them at an optimal level. When we make vitamin D in the skin, or obtain it from food and supplements, our body stores the vitamin D within the fat cells, to be used at a later date. Once the fat cells are saturated (or full) of vitamin D, then blood serum levels of 25(OH)D begin to rise to adequate levels. As illustrated in *Chapter 4: A Cellular Explanation*, 25(OH)D is the precursor to the active form and the hormone that is measured in our blood to determine if we have a healthy level of vitamin D in our body.

If you have a vitamin D deficiency, regardless of your weight, it will take some time to raise your serum levels of 25(OH)D to a healthy level. However, if you are overweight, it will take quite a bit longer to reach optimal vitamin D levels in your body because the fat cells will need to be saturated before your blood levels rise to optimal levels.

The good news is that when you have healthy vitamin D levels in your body, you're weight will typically decrease. Have you ever wondered why you were slimmer in the summer and heavier in the winter? There is a direct correlation between weight and vitamin D. With all things considered, people who live in areas that are sunny year round are overall lighter then those who live in areas that experience the four seasons. Obviously there are a great many factors that influence body type and weight, such as family history (genetics), eating habits, emotional eating, exercise routines, disabilities/injures, medications, metabolism, etc., but we do know that having optimal vitamin D levels will help every facet of your body's health, including its weight.

What about my lifestyle?

Assuming adequate sunlight, how you spend your time will greatly influence your vitamin D levels.

Clothing and sunscreen both block UVB rays from synthesizing vitamin D in the skin. In fact, studies have shown that Middle Eastern women are particularly at risk for being deficient because they are covered head to toe in fabric.

Do you work or spend long hours indoors? Is your sun exposure limited to walking back and forth to your car? Unfortunately, drive time cannot be counted toward getting your daily dose of vitamin D. Although the sun warms us through the glass, glass blocks out all UVB rays.

If you work outdoors year round it's likely that you are receiving enough sunlight for sufficient levels, however, care should be taken to avoid non-melanoma skin cancers. You can do this by applying sunscreen or clothing after you've obtained your daily dose of sunlight.

Behavior patterns greatly govern your vitamin D levels because ultimately, it's your choice to spend time in the sun or not. When considering ways to keep healthy levels of vitamin D in your body, please consider your behavior. While some behavior can be modified, such as applying sunscreen after sufficient sun exposure, if your habits or rituals keep you covered from the sun, please supplement! It's your way of providing your body with the necessary support to protect against illnesses and disease.

Chapter 6: Finding your optimal dose

"Because vitamin D is so cheap and so clearly reduces all-cause mortality, I can say this with great certainty: Vitamin D represents the single most cost-effective medical intervention in the United States."

Dr. Greg Plotnikoff, Medical Director
Penny George Institute of Health and Healing, Abbott Northwestern Hospital
in Minneapolis

At this point you may be concerned that you have a vitamin D deficiency. How do you find out and what do you do about it?

First things first: Your starting point

The first step is to find out your vitamin D status. This is done through a blood test for serum 25-hydroxy-D, otherwise known as 25(OH)D. This is a standard test done through your physician and is often times covered by insurance. There are also some mail-in tests available through the internet and one recommended by the Vitamin D Council.

The test directly measures circulating 25(OH)D levels in your blood, whether you obtain your vitamin D from the sun, diet or supplementation. In contrast, the active form of vitamin D, $1,25(OH)_2D$, is not a reliable measurement of your sufficiency and therefore is not recommended. It's also important to have your physician obtain serum levels during the dark/cold months and again during the summer months.

After an initial test to establish a baseline, and after beginning supplementation it is a good idea to recheck your serum levels again in 8-12 weeks. It can actually take as long as 8-12 weeks, if not longer, for tissue saturation. If you recall from chapter 5, tissue saturation is the process by where the fats cells become saturated with vitamin D before there is a measurable increase in the blood level vitamin D. If your vitamin D levels are low when you begin this process and/or you are overweight, give yourself time and stay consistent with your sun exposure or supplementation. It will naturally take quite a few months to reach protective serum levels.

I also recommend having your serum levels re-measured after another 16 weeks and again when the seasons change. It is crucial to stay 'optimal' and to not accumulate and cause vitamin D intoxication (over 150 ng/ml).

Acquiring this baseline serum level along with considering personal and environmental factors will give you and your physician enough information on how to help you reach optimal vitamin D level. Careful evaluation of these additional factors is the second step on the way to vitamin D sufficiency. A detailed look at these factors are found in *Chapter 5: What's blocking your sun*, and are summarized below.

Personal and environmental determinates

With the guidance of your physician, evaluate your personal and environmental factors and adjust your vitamin D dose and sun exposure as necessary.

> Personal determinates
> a. Skin color
> b. Body fat
> c. Dietary intake of vitamin D rich foods
> d. Kidney or liver disease
> e. Drug interactions
> f. Pregnancy or breastfeeding
> g. Age
> h. Clothing
> i. Use of sunscreen
>
> Environmental determinates
> a. Latitude
> b. Season
> c. How much time you spend in the sun
> d. Cloud cover
> e. Pollution
> f. Ozone and albedo (reflectivity).

Why is a physician necessary?

You may not think having your vitamin D serum levels checked is necessary before increasing your vitamin D supplementation. As you learned in the physiology chapter, the active form of vitamin D is intricately involved in the endocrine system and acts as a powerful hormone in your body. Having the guidance of a physician is important so that you don't create an imbalance in this system. Additionally, having a physician involved gives you the following advantages:

1. Serum levels are monitored for safety.
2. If you are extremely low and deficient a more aggressive vitamin D dosage can be implemented.
3. Your personal drug interactions can be monitored.
4. Health issues such as kidney and liver disease are accounted for.

What if I can't see my doctor?

The above situation is the ideal way to ascertain your required optimal dosing of vitamin D. However, if you are unable to receive medical guidance for some reason, a helpful suggestion is during the winter months to take between 2,000 – 5,000 units/day. In the summer, only supplement on days you are not out in the summertime sun.

What does my age have to do with it?

Age is an important factor and one that your physician needs to consider. Research has shown that if you are 49 years of age or older you are at a higher risk for vitamin D deficiency due to less sun exposure, less effective skin synthesis of vitamin D and a poor diet. When deficient levels of 25(OH)D exist, the body's main pathway for producing the active form (1,25(OH)2D) through the kidneys for regulating blood calcium levels is compromised. To keep this important system functioning, the parathyroid hormone (PTH) levels increase to mineralize the bones and release calcium into the blood.

Interestingly, this increase in PTH also keeps the active form of vitamin D at a normal level to regulate the blood calcium levels. This is one reason why serum levels of the active form are not an adequate indication of vitamin D health. In fact, these levels are often artificially high due to vitamin D deficiency and high PTH levels.

Dr. Malaban and others published an article in The Lancet in March of 1998 called <u>Redefining Vitamin D Insufficiency.</u> In this article he wrote that, "Therapy with 50,000 IU of oral vitamin D_2 weekly (by prescription only) for 8 weeks along with supplemental calcium, safely and effectively corrects secondary hyperparathyroidism, potentially leading to decreased fracture risk in the elderly."

What foods contain vitamin D?

Research has shown us that our vitamin D status is compromised and we often become deficient when we live at higher latitudes and the UVB rays from the sun are not available. As a result, dietary sources and supplementation have become important adjuncts for obtaining vitamin D.

Only a limited number of foods naturally contain natural vitamin D_3 (cholecalciferol). Contrastingly, vitamin D_2 (ergocalciferol) is present in some food sources such as mushrooms. Vitamin D_3 is the preferred source as it is absorbed much more efficiently in the intestines then vitamin D_2 and lasts approximately 10 times longer in the serum form.

Until recently, fortified foods were exclusively in the form of vitamin D_2. A gradual change to vitamin D_3 fortification has been adopted due to current research which shows the higher effectiveness of absorption, conversion and longevity of vitamin D_3.

The relatively short list of foods containing vitamin D, taken from vitamin D expert Dr. Holick's research paper, Vitamin D Deficiency printed in the New England Journal of Medicine, July 2007

Natural Sources	Vitamin D content
Salmon	
Fresh, wild (3.5 oz)	About 600 – 1,000 IU of vitamin D_3
Fresh, farmed (3.5 oz)	About 100-250 IU of vitamin D_3 or D_2
Canned (3.5 oz)	About 300-600 IU of vitamin D_3
Sardines	About 300 IU of vitamin D_3
Mackerel, canned	About 250 IU of vitamin D_3
Tuna, canned (3.6 oz)	About 230 IU of vitamin D_3
Cod liver oil (1 tsp)	About 400-1,000 IU of vitamin D_3
Shitake mushrooms	
Fresh (3.5 oz)	About 100 IU of vitamin D_2
Sun-dried (3.5 oz)	About 1,600 IU of vitamin D_2
Egg yolk	About 20 IU of vitamin D_3 or D_2

Fortified Foods	Vitamin D content
Fortified Milk	About 100 IU/8 oz, usually vitamin D_3
Fortified Orange juice	About 100 IU/8 oz, vitamin D_3
Fortified Infant formulas	About 100 IU/8 oz, vitamin D_3
Fortified Yogurts	About 100 IU/8 oz, usually vitamin D_3
Fortified Butter	About 50 IU/3.5 oz, usually vitamin D_3
Fortified Margarine	About 430 IU/3.5 oz, usually vitamin D_3
Fortified Cheeses	About 100 IU/3 oz, usually vitamin D_3
Fortified Breakfast cereals	About 100 IU/serving, usually vitamin D_3

Will eating foods with natural or fortified vitamin D increase my vitamin D levels sufficiently?

Unfortunately not. As you can from the list above, there are relatively few foods which contain vitamin D. Since most contain minimal amounts of vitamin D, and those like salmon are not consumed daily, there is a negligible effect on vitamin D serum levels.

What about Calcium?

Calcium levels are tied closely to vitamin D levels. Have you physician recommend a calcium supplement to take with your vitamin D supplement. If you are taking a calcium/magnesium supplement do not take it at the same time as your vitamin D supplement. Vitamin D and magnesium should not be taken at the same time.

When should I take my vitamin D supplement?

Always take your vitamin D with food, since it's an oil soluble vitamin. Consider taking it at a fatty meal along with calcium as well (unless it's a cal/mag supplement —see above). Vitamin D has a sedentary effect, therefore, consider taking it at dinnertime.

What drug interactions do I need to consider?

Most herbs and supplements have not been tested thoroughly for interactions with other herbs, supplements, drugs or foods. The following list of interactions are based on reports in scientific publications, or laboratory experiments. Always read product labels. If you have a medical condition or are taking prescription medication, herbs or supplements you should consult with a physician before initiating vitamin D therapy.

Antiseizure drugs: may decrease vitamin D levels due to their induction of liver enzymes which accelerate the conversion of vitamin D to inactive metabolites.

Cholestyramine/colestipol: inhibit intestinal absorption of vitamin D. Be advised to allow as much time as possible between the ingestion of these drugs and vitamin D.

Corticosteriods: can cause osteoporosis and calcium depletion with long-term administration. This situation creates a greater need for both supplemental calcium and vitamin D.

<u>Digoxin</u>: vitamin D should be used cautiously here since it may cause hypercalcemia, which may precipitate abnormal heart rhythms.

<u>Orlistat</u>: Can reduce vitamin D levels. Consider taking vitamin D or other fat-soluble vitamins at least 2 hours before or after Orlistat, but always with food.

<u>Rifampin</u>: increases vitamin D metabolism and so reduces vitamin D blood levels. Check serum levels regularly and dose accordingly.

<u>Stimulant laxatives</u>: Reduces dietary vitamin D absorption.

<u>Thiazide diuretics</u>: the concurrent use of thiazide (HCTZ) and vitamin D to hypoparathyroid patients may cause hypercalcemia, which may be transient or may require discontinuation of vitamin D.

Are there any nutritional interactions?

<u>Vitamin A</u>: Do not take with vitamin D since they are antagonistic supplements.

<u>Magnesium</u>: Do not take with vitamin D since they are antagonistic supplements.

I'm pregnant, what do I need to consider?

During pregnancy the recommended adequate intake (AI) for pregnant women is the same as for non-pregnant women. However, researchers have suggested that requirements during pregnancy are much greater than these amounts. Make certain your physician regularly evaluates your vitamin D status while pregnant and optimizes your serum 25(OH)D levels to ensure proper fetal brain development.

What about breastfed and formula fed babies?

Vitamin D is most always deficient in maternal milk. To prevent deficiency and rickets in exclusively breastfed and formulated infants, supplementation needs to be considered. For breast fed infants, having the mothers serum levels checked is important. Start with a baseline then recheck in 4-6 weeks after vitamin D supplementation has started. If mom's level is optimal (50-60 ng/ml) while breast feeding, the baby should be receiving an optimal amount as well. Also, consider the amount of vitamin D production you may be receiving from outdoors (without sunscreen) if it is summer outside. You may need much less supplementing if this is the case.

Formula fed infants receive approximately 400 IU of vitamin D/day with their milk. See the list below for supplementation recommendations by the vitamin D experts for formula fed babies.

How much vitamin D does my child need?

According to Dr. Cannell and other experts at the vitamin D council, the rise in childhood illness and autism has a direct link to vitamin D deficiency. They have proposed vitamin D supplementation for ages 0-10 that will create a much healthier population and hopefully halt and reverse the rise in autism, asthma and diabetes type 1 in children.

Breast fed babies: 1,000 IU/day. Follow this supplementation recommendation unless the mother is vitamin D sufficient, getting plenty of sunlight or taking 4,000-6,000 IU/day

Formula fed babies: 600 IU/day. There is no need to supplement on days your child is getting plenty of sunshine (without sunscreen). Avoid sunburns by applying sunscreen or clothing before the skin begins to redden. Supplement in the wintertime unless you live below 40° latitude.

Children ages 1-3 years: 2,000 IU/day. No need to supplement during the summertime when your child is getting his or her daily dose of sunshine. Avoid sunburns by applying sunscreen or clothing before the skin begins to redden. Supplement in the wintertime unless you live below 40° latitude.

Children ages 4-10 years: 3,000 IU/day. No need to supplement during the summertime when your child is getting his or her daily dose of sunshine. Avoid sunburns by applying sunscreen or clothing before the skin begins to redden. Supplement in the wintertime unless you live below 40° latitude.

How pure is my vitamin D supplement?

Upon researching the top health food store brands, so far none has checked out to utilize the pure vitamin D. Professional brands however, do use the purest vitamin D available. These brands are commonly available through your naturopathic physician and possibly online. One particularly good brand is Thorne Research. Thorne manufactures their own

supplements with very strict quality control standards. Upon investigation we found they also put no unhealthy fillers in their products. We recommend you check out your brand carefully before purchase. Since I am
a physician who constantly measures my patient's serum vitamin D levels,
I use a higher dose of D from Thorne or I frequently utilize 'D' drops from
Biotics.

In my practice, after measuring hundreds of patient's serum levels, I have
concluded that the liquid form (drops or capsules) is more highly effective.
The dry form doesn't seem to increase serum levels as quickly and may be
more difficult to digest, especially if there is no fat around for it to get
absorbed with.

What does the FDA have to say?

The US Food and Drug Administration (FDA) does not strictly regulate
herbs and supplements. Therefore, there is no guarantee of purity,
strength or safety of products. Effects may vary. If you have a medical
condition or are taking other drugs, herbs or supplements, you should
seek out a licensed physician before initiating a new therapy, such as vitamin D. Consult a physician immediately if you experience any side
effects.

Safety Issues - side effects and warnings

Let's say it's a sunny day. Your body is soaking in rays of sunshine and
making vitamin D. As, your skin makes pre-vitamin D, its estimated that
you'll produce approximately 15,000 IU of vitamin D_3 in as little as 30 minutes depending on skin type. Considering these are the numbers produced daily when we're in the sun, it is poorly founded that potential
overdoses may occur with supplements. In fact, the researcher Dr. Vieth,
believes people need 4,000 – 10,000 IU of vitamin D daily and that the
toxic side effects are not a concern until 40,000 IU a day are continued for
a period of time. The dose of 4,000-10,000 IU per day needs to be monitored by your physician by regularly checking your serum 25(OH)D levels.

Vitamin D from the sun as well as diet and supplement are generally well
tolerated. However, it is important to consider those at risk of developing toxicity. Vitamin D toxicity can result from regular excess intake of this
vitamin and may lead to hypercalcemia and excess bone loss. People at
increased risk for developing toxicity include those with hyperparathyroidism, sarcoidosis, kidney disease, tuberculosis or histoplasmosis.

Chronically high blood calcium levels may lead to serious complications and should be managed by a doctor. Symptoms of high blood calcium levels may include: nausea, vomiting, anorexia followed by excess thirst, excess urination, weakness, fatigue, somnolence, headache, dry mouth, metallic taste, vertigo, tinnitus and ataxia (unsteadiness), kidney dysfunction and calcium deposition in different organs may occur. Treatment involves physician supervision; halting all vitamin D and calcium. Frequent monitoring of calcium levels is imperative until they normalize again.

Those at risk of toxic levels of vitamin D:

It is critically important for a physician to monitor your vitamin D status before beginning any regime if you have any of the following:

Hyperparathyroidism
Histoplasmosis
Granulomatous diseases
Kidney stones
Kidney disease
Sarcoidosis
Tuberculosis

People at risk for vitamin D deficiency:

If you fall into any of the following categories, or have any of the following diseases or conditions, you may be vitamin D deficient. Please visit you physician to ascertain your current serum level and get an optimal dose of vitamin D.

At risk catagories
Vegan
Elderly, over 49
Pregnant
Breastfeeding
Infant/toddler
Adolescent
Nursing home residents
Those living at Northern latitudes

Diseases and conditions:

All chronic degenerative disorders
All cancer patients
All auto-immune disorders
Osteoporosis

Chapter 7: Shedding Light on Skin Health and Skin Cancer

"No other method to prevent cancer has been identified that has such a powerful impact."

Dr. Cedric Garland. Vitamin D Expert

Skin is the largest organ of the body. Most of us don't think of the skin as an organ. When we think of body organs the heart, lungs, liver or kidneys may spring to mind. We have a number of internal organs and one very large and vital external organ, the skin.

Our skin is remarkable. It responds immediately to injuries by bringing a blood supply of nutrients to heal the affected area. It needs to heal and do it quickly because it has a number of important jobs to do. First off, it's the first line of defense against the outside world. We intuitively know this because whenever we sustain a cut, we immediately bandage our skin. Bacteria and viruses are all around us and our skin does a fabulous job of protecting us from this unseen world. But when we have any kind of open wound, those microbes can enter our skin and possibly our body. By bandaging the skin, we are providing a protective covering while the skin works to heal itself.

The skin also regulates our body temperature, retains water, provides a cocoon to protect our vital organs, synthesizes vitamin D, produces melanin and has its own immune system and barrier 'acid mantle' to protect against bacteria.

Skin is composed of three distinct layers. The top layer is called the epidermis. The epidermis is subdivided into five layers with a number of specialized cells. It is also the thinnest layer of our skin. The second layer is called the dermis. The dermis is thicker and filled with blood vessels, glands, nerve endings and hair follicles. It also houses the structural elements of connective tissue and imparts elasticity. The third layer has more connective tissue, larger blood vessels, more nerves and a higher amount of fat which is used to regulate the temperature of our skin and body.

Where in the skin is vitamin D made?

Vitamin D is made in the top layer of our skin, the epidermis. It all starts when a photon of UVB radiation hits a cellular molecule called 7DHC, or 7-dihydroxyvitmain D. This reaction initiates a photoisomerization within the cell to produce pre-vitamin D. This is the first step in the process of making vitamin D. The entire process is detailed in *Chapter 4: A Cellular Explanation.*

Where does getting a tan come into all this?

But what else happens when we are exposed to sunlight? The epidermis houses another specialized cell called a melanocyte. The melanocyte competes with 7DHC for sunlight. When an inactive melanocyte encounters UVB radiation it produces melanin. If we have lighter skin, we experience this reaction as a tan, but its purpose is to produce melanin which protects the cells from damage due to overexposure to the sun.

Your melanocytes are showing

Everyone has melanocytes in their epidermis. It's interesting to learn that it isn't that people with darker skin have more melanocytes than people with lighter skin. No, we all have a relatively equal numbers of these cells. Where we get the variance in skin pigmentation is from the activity level within these cells. People with highly active melanocytes produce melanin constantly and have the darkest skin tones. People with relatively inactive melanocytes have the lightest skin tone. In between there lies a wide range of melanocyte activity and resulting skin tones.

The evolution of skin tones

Melanocyte activity has its roots in evolution. Our ancestors living closest to the equator were subject to long hours under strong sunlight. They evolved to have highly active melanocytes that were constantly producing melanin. When melanin is active in the cell, it acts like natural sunblock, reflecting the radiation away from us and thereby protecting the cellular DNA from being damaged. As a result, people with darker skin can tolerate long periods of time under direct sunlight without experiencing harmful effects.

Our ancestors living further north or south of the equator didn't need to evolve highly active melanocytes because the sun was less intense and less available. They even had months each year where usable sunlight for vitamin D production was not available.

When we understand how skin developed based on evolution, we can see why lighter skin needs less exposure time to make vitamin D than darker skin. It was an evolutionary need for our ancestors living north and south of the equator to adapt and utilize available sunlight to quickly make vitamin D.

You will also notice evolutionarily, that skin tones follow the gradient of the earth; darkest at the center and gradually decreasing in tone the further you rise or fall from that point.

What's your skin tone?

Researchers have subdivided skin into 6 tones.

Type I	Translucent skin. Always burn. Never tan
Type 2	Fair skin. Burn easily. Rarely tan.
Type 3	Light skin. Tans gradually. Occasionally burn.
Type 4	Medium skin. Always Tan. Rarely burn.
Type 5	Medium to dark skin. Seldom burn. Always tan.
Type 6	Blue-black skin. Never burn. Tan darkly

People with type I skin tones never tan. They are typically people with albino skin or very light skinned and redheaded. These people always burn and are in the highest risk group for developing skin cancer. Type 1 and type 2 skin tones have recently been shown to be deficient in vitamin D, despite their relatively fast production of vitamin D. This could be due to their avoidance of the sun and fear of sunburns.

People with medium to dark skin tones who live at Northern latitudes, who do not supplement with vitamin D and/or who do not get enough sunlight exposure are at a high risk for vitamin D deficiency. This is due to the longer period of time required in the sunlight to synthesize vitamin D in the skin.

What length of time should I expose my skin to sunlight?

To make vitamin D in our skin we need to expose it to UVB radiation. UVB radiation is found in sunlight and has been bottled for us in tanning booths. We now understand the purpose of melanin and how it effectively blocks sunlight from damaging our skin. And we also know that melanin competes with cells containing 7DHC which produce pre-vitamin D. Suffice to say, when our skin is darker we will need more time in the sun to make vitamin D, then if our skin is lighter.

So, how much time is that? Dr. Holick, the leading expert on vitamin D advocates building vitamin D levels from sunlight exposure. Sunlight is free and our skin is highly effective at making vitamin D. There is also no risk of vitamin D toxicity when synthesized by the skin.

Since research has shown the sun to be the 'optimal' method of acquiring vitamin D, consider sun tanning, but wisely and with the following suggestions:

- Stay in the sun long enough to synthesize at least your minimum dose, but stop before your maximum dose. You maximum dose is the time required for your skin to turn slightly pink under strong sunlight. (Any sign of pink means the skin is beginning to burn).
- Cover up with clothing or sunscreen if you plan on staying in the sun longer.
- Avoid any chance of sunburn. Sunburns early in life are associated with later development of melanoma.

If you are not outside during the hottest part of the day, the sun is less intense and you will be able to stay in sun longer without burning. Please use the sun wisely and be safe. By exposing your skin to the sun to make vitamin D and covering up afterward to protect your skin from burning, you will be harnessing all the beneficial effects without risking the development of any of the skin cancers.

What is cancer?

Cancer is the result of a normal body process behaving abnormally. In healthy tissue, our cells grow by dividing themselves. Cancer occurs when this process of cell growth by division happens too quickly. The cells begin multiplying out of control and the result is lots of extra cells in the form of tumors and growths. When this occurs in our skin it's called skin cancer.

Cancer is a frightening word. There are few other words that scare us as much. If we were each diagnosed with cancer this instant, I bet the first thing we'd want to know is if we'd survive. What are our chances? What we don't always realize however, is there are lots of cancers that are very treatable and rarely fatal. The non-melanoma skin cancers fall into this category.

Understanding Skin Cancer

Non-melanoma skin cancers are the most common of all skin cancers. Basal Cell Carcinoma (BCC) is the most common type, affecting approximately 1 million people each year. Squamous Cell Carcinoma (SCC) is the second most common with approximately 250,000 new cases each year. Of these 1,250,000 new cases each year, only 0.3% result in fatality. While these survival statistics are very good, it's important to know more about these types of cancers and catch them early. As with all cancers, the earlier they are detected the better.

Basal Cell Carcinoma - BCC

Basal cell carcinoma occurs in the basal cells of the epidermis. This type of cancer is found on the areas that were exposed to the sun such as the face, ears, nose and shoulders. Painful sunburns are associated with the development of basal cell carcinoma, whereas, regular, moderate sun exposure is much less implicated as a cause in their development. In other words, mild to moderate skin exposure may actually protect you from developing basal cell carcinoma. This is due to the steady progression of melanin production protecting your skin from harsh sun rays.

Any type of sunburn negates the protective effects of melanin and might actually cause an immunosuppressive effect. By suppressing the skin's immune system by getting a sunburn - your chances of developing skin cancer rises.

Squamous Cell Carcinoma - SCC

Squamous Cell Carcinoma also occurs in the epidermis. However, different from BCC, squamous cell carcinoma is often the result of chronic overexposure to the sun. While sunburns are implicated in all types of skin cancers, SCC's are typically caused by long-term overexposure. Squamous cell carcinoma, like BCC's, also occur on areas of the skin that are most frequently exposed to the sun. Squamous cell carcinoma's are typically found on the face, neck, bald scalps, hands, shoulders, arms and back. The rim of the ear and the lower lip are especially vulnerable to developing squamous cell carcinoma.

Actinic Keratosis - AK

Actinic Keratosis, or sometimes called AK's were typically thought of as 'pre' skin cancer. However, AK's are now considered to be cutaneous squamous cell carcinoma *in situ* (before it metastasizes -spreads) AK's are more frequent in men, sun sensitive individuals exposed to chronic sun and in people who have a history of sunburns. AK's occur when there is a change in the cells of the epidermis. This change can be seen as rough white, red or brown scaly patches and they typically occur on areas that are exposed to the sun.

Malignant Melanoma

Malignant melanoma is the most serious of all skin cancers. They are the least common, affecting about 60,000 people a year, but with a fatality of approximately 8,000. This represents a 13% fatality rate and 133 times greater risk of dying than from both non-melanoma skin cancers combined.

There is hopeful news however. The Skin Cancer Foundation has reported that even with malignant melanoma, the most serious skin cancer, if it is caught early enough, the survival rate is 100%. The above fatalities occur when melanoma goes undetected.

Melanoma is highly associated with bad sunburns during childhood. If you experienced blistering sunburns during early childhood and you have type 1 or 2 skin tones you have the highest risk for developing malignant melanoma later in life. Screen your skin by conducting a self examination at least every 6 months and report any abnormalities to your physician.

When conducting a self examination of your skin it's important to look at your whole body. Malignant melanoma's, unlike basal and squamous cell carcinoma's are not usually found on areas exposed to the sun. **Melanoma's commonly appear on an area of the body which have never seen the sun!** Melanoma's originate in the melanocytes, the cells that produce melanin. When melanoma's develop they are typically brown or black. However, there are cases of them being skin colored, pink, purple, blue and white.

Risk factors for developing melanoma

    a. Blistering sunburns in early childhood.
    b. People with type 1 or 2 skin tones and who've experienced sunburns.

c. The number of moles on your body. The more moles you have the higher your risk. People with type 1 skin tones often times have a lot of moles.
d. A family history of melanoma.
e. There is also a study that showed an increased incidence of malignant melanoma with decreasing latitude toward the equator. The closer you live to the equator, the higher your chances are for getting sunburned, which puts you at higher risk for developing melanoma.

Will using sunscreens now protect me from melanoma?

No. Unfortunately, if you've experienced sunburns at any time in your life and especially in childhood, you are at risk for developing melanoma. A study was published in 1995 that actually showed an increased risk of developing melanoma after sunscreen use. People often begin using sunscreen to avoid experiencing another sunburn, which is the major factor in developing malignant melanoma. Strict use of sunscreen can increase the risk of this deadly cancer, because it lowers vitamin D levels and the anti-cancer effect of vitamin D is lost.

Sun exposure helps malignant melanoma?

Regular-less-intense exposure to the sun is not a risk factor for developing malignant melanoma. On the contrary, this type of sun exposure has been shown to be protective. Scientist's have also found that sun exposure is associated with a relatively favorable prognosis and increased survival rates in various malignancies including malignant melanoma. This is because of the health benefits we get from the sun. This isn't surprising since vitamin D is the best cancer fighter of all.

Hopefully soon, dermatologists and other clinicians will recognize the compelling evidence, statistics and benefits of regular, moderate and less intense exposure to the UVB rays of the sun and that these far outweigh its mutagenic effects.

Why is my skin prematurely aging when I've been using sunscreen?

When sunscreens first hit the market they were designed to block the burning rays of the sun, the UVB rays. UVA rays are not associated with skin cancer as they do not cause sunburns. Because UVA rays bring about a deeper and longer lasting tan they were not part of early sunscreen formulations.

Let's say you applied a strong SPF sunscreen with UVB protection and you stayed in the sun all day. You didn't burn, but the entire day you were absorbing UVA rays. You were in fact getting a high dose of UVA rays because you were staying outside longer than you would have if you didn't have on sunscreen. Unfortunately, UVA rays have been found to be a major cause of skin aging. They penetrate right through the epidermis (the top layer) and into the dermis layer of skin where they cause damage. The dermis layer is where we have our collagen and elasticity. By exposing our skin to large quantities of UVA rays, we inadvertently caused our skin to prematurely age.

Most sunscreens on the market today are formulated to protect against UVA and UVB rays. UVB affects skin cancer development (predominantly in the epidermis) and UVA causes the deeper (dermis) skin aging. Since both UVA and UVB can induce structural damage to DNA, they both can damage the skin.

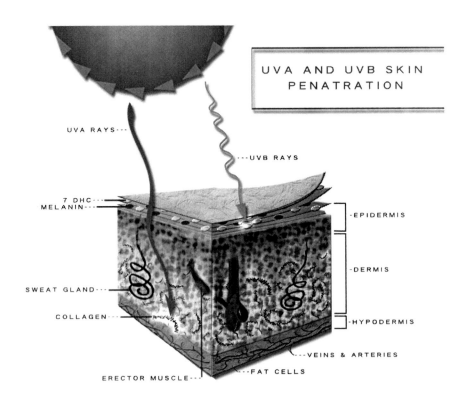

A word about tanning beds

I recently went to my local tanning salon and the girls at the front desk were recommending the higher pressure tanning beds. When I said I was only there for the vitamin D, they still recommended the other beds over the conventional tanning bed and told me I could make vitamin D from the higher pressure tanning beds. They were taught that the burning rays were the UVB rays and the tanning rays were the UVA rays. This is correct in that over exposure to UVB will burn your skin and UVA rays penetrate deeper and give you a longer lasting tan. What is misleading to many people is that they are getting the beneficial effects of the sun by making vitamin D in their skin from the UVA rays. These rays are longer and reach into the skin deeper. They are not capable or responsible for making pre-vitamin D in your skin. I recommend using a conventional tanning bed if you are not able to get your vitamin D from the natural sunlight. If you are tanning, do so safely and avoid burning.

And remember, those UVA rays are the ones that are damaging the collagen and elasticity of your skin. By using the higher pressure tanning beds, you are not only paying more money, you are speeding up the skin aging process and get none of the beneficial effects of vitamin D production.

What's your wavelength good buddy?

UVA (320nm-400nm)

- Longer wavelength penetrates into dermal layer of the skin
- Aging of skin – damage to connective tissue and elasticity
- Longer lasting tan

UVB (280nm - 320nm)

- Shorter wavelength penetrates epidermal layer of skin
- Pre-vitamin D production = significant health benefits and vitality
- Regular exposure without sunburn increases protection from cancers including skin cancer
- Overexposure resulting in sunburns increases risk of skin cancer. While afflicted with a sunburn, the skin cannot produce pre-vitamin D.

My suggestion

All of us want to avoid skin cancer and any other cancer for that matter. With the overwhelming protective benefits from vitamin D, especially the cancer fighting benefits, I feel it's critical to keep your vitamin D levels optimal. When it comes to skin cancer it's a classic catch 22 – the same sun which adds years to your life can also cause extensive damage to your skin. A great solution is to absorb just the right amount and then cover up!

Chapter 8: Sunscreen 101

> "Poisoning your body with toxic sunscreen chemicals while block-ing nourishing sunlight that generates vitamin D (which reduces overall cancer risk by 50%) is nothing short of health lunacy."
>
> Mike Adams, Consumer Health Advocate

We have been scared out of the sun for fear of skin cancers and aging for several years now. And with all the intense campaigning of strict 'no sun' recommendations; the sunscreen companies are flourishing but our health is certainly not! Even in Northern latitudes, women are repri-manded by their dermatologists and/or aestheticians to wear sunscreens even in cloudy weather.

There has to be a 'middle path' for people to have moderate sun exposure and skin protection simultaneously. I believe the best way to navigate this 'middle path' is best done through education. If you know what you're dealing with, you'll know how to make informed decisions.

Welcome to Sunscreen 101!

Sunscreen use can increase your risk of acquiring deadly cancers

When sunscreens are used religiously - that is applying sunscreen to your skin whenever you're in the sun – you are preventing sunlight the oppor-tunity of producing vitamin D in your skin, and are thereby thwarting the first step in a series that will protect you from a variety of diseases includ-ing some serious cancers! How is that possible? Here it is in a nut shell:

 a. Sunlight is our main source of vitamin D.
 b. Healthy levels of vitamin D protect the body from serious diseases such as breast cancer, prostate cancer, ovarian cancer, colon can-cer – in fact many different cancers.
 c. By cutting off your main supply of vitamin D by from overly con-scious sunscreen use it's likely your vitamin D levels are deficient.
 d. Vitamin D deficiency is associated with a much higher risk of can-cer, auto-immune diseases and heart disease.

What are carcinogens and why are they in my sunscreen?

Sunscreens have been evaluated for effectiveness as well as their chemi-cal contents. Unfortunately, some sunscreens contain chemicals which cause cancer and are known as carcinogens. Since most of us are applying sunscreen with the purpose to protect our skin from cancer, it seems ironic that this very substance may 'double' as a carcinogen. So, not only does the religious use of sunscreens increase our risk of cancer because it prevents us from having the protective effects of healthy vitamin D levels, but many also contain deleterious chemicals which can cause cancer!

In 2009, the Environmental Working Group (EWG) conducted a sunscreen investigation analyzing 500 different name brand sunscreens. They found that, "3 of 5 don't protect skin from sun damage or contain hazardous chemicals, or both."

Here is a list of the common chemicals found in sunscreens (listed compiled by Green Living Tips at www.greenlivingtips.com). Please read the label and choose a 'safe' sunscreen that does not contain carcinogens!

Aminobenzoic acid - possible carcinogen may be implicated in cardiovascular disease.
Avobenzone - possible carcinogen
Cinoxate - some evidence of skin toxicity
Dioxybenzone - strong evidence of skin toxicity and possible carcinogen; hormone disruptor and has been found in waterways, soil and air. Has been shown to have a "gender bender" effect in animals
Diazolidinyl urea - possible carcinogen, endocrine, central nervous system and brain effects, skin toxicity and compromises the immune system
Ecamsule - may be carcinogenic
Homosalate - endocrine disruption
Methylparaben - interferes with genes
Octocrylene - found to be persistent and bioaccumulative in wildlife, liver issues and possible carcinogen
Octyl methoxycinnamate - accumulates in the body, may disrupt liver and is a possible carcinogen
Octyl salicylate - broad systemic effects in animals at moderate doses
Oxybenzone - possible carcinogen and contributor to vascular disease, may affect the brain and nervous system in animals
Padimate O - suspected carcinogen
Phenylbenzimidazole - possible carcinogen
Phenoxyethanol - irritant, possible carcinogen, endocrine disruption
Sulisobenzone - strong evidence of skin toxicity, affects sense organs in animals

What sunscreens are safe?

The website of the Environmental Working Group (EWG) lists the best easy-to-find sunscreens. For updates you can visit them at www.ewg.org or at www.cosmeticdatabase.com. For 2009, their list includes the brands: California baby, Mustela, Mission Skincare, Neutrogena, Blue Lizard, Jason Natural, Earth's Best, Solar Sense, CVS and Coppertone Water BABIES (Pure&Simple).

How can I use my sunscreen wisely?

After you've exposed your skin to the sunlight for the recommended time needed for vitamin D production to occur (10 minutes or longer depending on your skin type) apply a generous amount of 'safe' sunscreen for the duration of your time in the sun and/or cover up with clothing and hats. This will ensure you receive your optimal vitamin D (UVB) dose and you'll be protecting you skin from any chance of sunburn, therefore reducing your risk of skin cancer and skin damage caused by UVA rays.

If you are particularly concerned with protecting your face from prematurely aging, apply a sunscreen to your face daily that blocks UVA radiation. You'll be able to get your vitamin D produced in other areas of exposed skin, such as your legs and arms.

Most importantly, when you are ready to apply your sunscreen you must use a generous amount in order for it to be effective! Many people don't use enough and experience sunburns in the places they missed or where the coverage was not great enough. Remember, any sunburn will increase your chances for melanoma and skin damage.

What is PABA and why do sunscreens state that they are PABA-Free?

PABA is para-aminobenzoic acid and was once a very popular sunscreen ingredient that fell out of favor with manufacturers because of problems with allergic dermatitis and/or photosensitivity. This "PABA-Free" marketing claim is nearly all meaningless since virtually most sunscreens are devoid of PABA at this time. A derivative of PABA called Padimate O is still used however, and can be found in sunscreens which are PABA-Free. Padimate O appears to be safer than PABA, but still shares some similar health concerns as its parent chemical and is a possible carcinogen.

How safe are sunscreens containing nano particles?

Many zinc and titanium sunscreen products contain nano particles, even when they are not on the label. Nano size particles are more easily absorbed by the epidermis because of their small size, hence there are some concerns over toxicity. Oddly enough, when all the factors were weighed with respect to sunscreen safety, the Environmental Working Group found that many zinc and titanium containing sunscreens were found to be the safest and most effective on the market.

One study showed that consumers who used sunscreens without zinc and titanium were likely exposed to more UV radiation and greater numbers of hazardous ingredients than consumers who rely on zinc and titanium for sun protection. Skin Deep, a cosmetic safety database, found that consumers using sunscreens without zinc and titanium are exposed to an average of 20% more UVA radiation. This increased UVA exposure damages the skin causing premature aging, wrinkling and UVA induced immune system damage.

In these same sunscreens, those without zinc and titanium, Skin Deep found at least four high hazard ingredients which are known or strongly suspicious carcinogens. They also contain more toxins on average in every major category of health harm considered: Cancer (10% more), birth defects and reproductive harm (40% more), neurotoxins (70% more) and chemicals that can damage the immune system (70% more).

Zinc Oxide and Titanium dioxide are stable compound that provide a broad spectrum UVA and UVB protection. The available studies consistently show very little or zero penetration of intact skin by these compounds; indicating that real world exposure to potential nano size particles in these products is likely very low, whereas the sun protection benefits are very high.

The Environmental Working Group's rating of zinc and titanium products states that they are among the safest and most effective sunscreens available in the US today.

Are there any other considerations when picking a sunscreen?

Yes. The EWG's 2009 report recommends avoiding spray-on and power sunscreens as inhaling the chemicals poses an added risk. Sunscreens with added bug-repellant also made the list of sunscreens to avoid as too much pesticide can enter your body through skin absorption.

What does SPF really mean?

SPF, or Sun Protection Factor is a measurement of time that will protect your skin from burning when you're in the sun. This amount of time is specific for each person as it is dependent on how long you can stay in the sun normally without turning pink. Let's say you can stay in the hot mid-day sun for 15 minutes without your skin reddening. If you apply a SPF of 8 this will increase your 15 minutes by eight times (15 x 8 = 120 minutes) allowing you to stay outdoors for 2 hours without skin reddening. If you apply a SPF 30 the calculation would be (15 x 30 = 450 minutes or 7.5 hours). This is only an estimate however, because skin type, activities (sweating/swimming), and intensity of the sun, all affect how much you need and how effective the sunscreen will be.

SPF ratings can also be confusing or misleading. The rating instructs you how to use the product to protect against sunburns caused by UVB radiation, but they say nothing about protection from UVA rays. It may be a sunscreen that blocks UVA and UVB, but how long can you stay in the sun without skin damage occurring? They don't tell us.

The SPF rating scale is not linear for high SFP's.

What does this mean? Well, an SPF 50 does not prevent burns 2/3 times longer than SPF 30. In fact, it blocks only 1.3% more UVB radiation. The FDA has suggested that the current testing methods may not be able to accurately determine SPF values for products containing SPF's over 15.

How high of a SPF should I use?

The American Cancer Society recommends that people use a sunscreen with an SPF of at least 15. Higher SPF's may give you more protection, but as a consumers you should know that once you reach SPF 30, there is not much difference between products with higher SPF values, except for a higher price!

What should I remember most about sunscreen?

1. Avoiding the sun at all costs by applying sunscreen whenever you are outdoors, increases your risk of developing diseases associ-

ated with vitamin D deficiency such as cancer, autoimmune diseases and heart failure.

2. Apply a safe sunscreen and/or clothing after you've gotten your daily dose of sunshine.
3. Avoid sunscreens containing hazardous chemicals and carcinogens which are highly toxic to your health.
4. Apply a UVA and UVB sunscreen product to protect against sunburns and skin aging.

Chapter 9: Are You Sad?

"The sun is the orchestra leader for the dance of life. Every living thing on earth vibrates to the energy of the sun, including people. For a long time people have been victims of a huge scam that made them think they were supposed to hide indoors or under a blanket of sunscreen while the rest of life basked in the glory of the sun. Now they are catching on that they too need the sun's life-giving force."

Barbara Minton, Natural Health Editor.

Sunlight not only affects our health in terms of vitamin D levels, but it is the sole regulator of our bodies sleep and wake cycles. These cycles are known as circadian rhythms and they fluctuate depending on the amount of light we are exposed to.

When fall descends on us and the hours of daylight begin to shorten, we may begin to feel a change in our overall energy level. We may find ourselves sleeping a little more in the winter or eating more comfort foods, rich in carbohydrates, and less fresh fruits and vegetables. It is normal for everyone to experience some variance in energy and mood within the seasons, but when it seriously impacts your ability to function and cope, there's a chemical imbalance happening that needs to be addressed.

What's happening to me?

Sunlight chemically stimulates the hypothalamus in our brains by entering through the retina of our eyes. The effect is a signal from the hypothalamus to the pineal gland telling it to stop producing melatonin (the chemical which makes us sluggish and sleepy) and start producing serotonin (the chemical that helps us wake up, feel alert and be happy). In some people reduced daylight hours causes a disturbance in melatonin and serotonin levels. This disturbance is a condition known as Seasonal Affective Disorder, or SAD.

Do you have SAD symptoms?

- Do you experience a depression that begins in the fall/winter and lasts through springtime?

- Are your typical symptoms of depression: negative-irrational thoughts, apathy and despair?
- Do you have a lack of motivation?
- Do you find yourself dragging through the day?
- Do you have unusual cravings for sweets and carbs?
- Do you overeat? Does this lead to weight gain?
- Do you feel anxious and irritable?
- Do you isolate or socially withdrawal?
- Do you have a low libido (low sex drive)?
- Are you moody?
- Do you have difficulty sleeping at night or have poor sleep habits?
- Do you sleep for unusually long hours?
- Are you overly active in the spring and summer?
- Do you get sick easily? Is your immune system weakened?

If you are experiencing more than a couple of the above symptoms, during the winter months or dark days, you are likely experiencing Seasonal Affective Disorder. But, don't worry, you are not alone. Millions of people every year are affected with SAD from October thru April. The good news is there are natural ways to combat this disorder without the use of anti-depressants. In fact, studies have shown that light therapies are more effective then antidepressants for treating SAD.

The chemicals

Reduced daylight hours means longer night time hours. This in turn increases production of melatonin, the chemical that makes us feel sluggish and tired and helps us go to sleep. In addition to shorter days, areas with dense cloud cover block out the sun making the daytime we do have even darker, which increases melatonin levels further.

The reduction in light, caused by shorter and/or dark days, does not give people with SAD enough 'cues' to awaken during the day. The low light decreases production of serotonin and since serotonin helps us feel happy and calm, its deficiency causes us to feel irritable and depressed. Low serotonin/high melatonin levels are the underlying cause of SAD. When these chemicals are out of balance there is an overall feeling of being groggy, fatigued, exhausted and sleepy throughout the day – it's as if the body can't wake up.

When spring and summer arrive, the days are longer and brighter which in turn enhances serotonin production and corrects the imbalance of high melatonin levels.

Seattle happens to be the epitome of a dark-cloudy city, at least from October till July 4th. SAD and depression run rampant in the Pacific Northwest; along with very high rates of breast cancer, MS, and all the other vitamin D deficiency diseases. Dark cloudy weather keeps vitamin D levels low, serotonin levels low and melatonin levels high.

My medical practice is in the Seattle area and I have personally noticed an appalling number of women on antidepressants. It is also fact, by the way, that women have more serotonin receptor sites than men, making them more vulnerable to deficiency states.

You may have been misdiagnosed

I've also noticed within my patient populous, that women placed on antidepressants, commonly still complain of lingering depression and fatigue. Upon further questioning, most of them still experience SAD symptoms. Unfortunately, many of these women were not properly diagnosed and treated. They were given the diagnosis of depression rather than Seasonal Affective Disorder (SAD). This may be hard to catch for clinicians in rainy areas because the symptoms of SAD can occur practically year round under dense cloud cover.

It is my recommendation that health practitioners, who practice in low-light areas like Seattle, check the serotonin, melatonin, thyroid and vitamin D levels of their depressed patient's. Correcting and optimizing these hormone and vitamin deficiencies must be made standard of care *before* hastily writing antidepressant prescriptions.

Most medical doctors (MD's) have very little experience with alternative medicine and its approach for looking at the underlying cause of disease. For example, when a woman visits her MD and complains of fatigue, an MD would run standard tests for iron and TSH. If these tests results are within the 'normal' range, she will commonly get labeled with 'depression' and walk out with a prescription for Prozac, Zoloft, Paxil or the newest incarnation of antidepressant.

Sunlight on the other hand affects our neuro-hormonal systems; raising serotonin levels and reducing melatonin levels, so that anxiety is replaced with calm and doom is replaced by cheerfulness. With melatonin in balance; daytime fatigue burns off and sleep at night becomes deep and restful again.

If you are currently misdiagnosed with depression and you actually have Seasonal Affective Disorder, you've likely been treated with antidepressants which may not be relieving your symptoms. SAD is a neuro-hormonal imbalance that can be treated naturally with nutrition and light therapy.

How do I find out if I was misdiagnosed?

Have your physician run the following tests to determine your correct diagnosis. If you know what you have, you'll know how to best treat it!

1. Serotonin
2. Melotonin
3. Thyroid (TSH and Free T3 and T4)
4. Vitamin D (25(OH)D)

SAD patients – don't wean yourself off antidepressants!

As a clinician, I never recommend anyone withdraw from their antidepressant by themselves. What I do recommend, is to first correct the underlying reason for the depression, such as high melatonin levels, and once you feel better, then gently and slowly wean off your medication, but ONLY under the supervision of your physician.

Depressed patients – don't stop taking your medication!

It is not recommended that you withdraw from your antidepressants at all if you have moderate clinical depression. You can still have your physician test your serotonin, melatonin, thyroid and vitamin D levels. If these are out of balance you will also benefit from the following therapies for SAD, but do not stop taking your medication!

What is a light box and how is that going to help?

Light boxes are small but powerful allies to combat SAD. They emit the full spectrum wavelength that simulates the brightest sunlight, that of solar noon. The light enters the retina of the eyes and which stimulates the production of serotonin and turns off the production of melatonin. In Dr. Holick's book, *The UV Advantage*, he explains that light boxes are designed to emit between 5,000 and 10,000 lux (a lux is light measurement – the same way a pound (lb) is a weight measurement). The typical bright lighting in an office only emits 500-700 lux which is only the strength of light at twilight. If a person with SAD is only exposed to light that is equivalent to early morning or late evening light, a time of day most of us are slower moving, their brains aren't stimulated enough to make the chemicals needed to completely wake up.

How and when do I use my light box?

There are light boxes on a timer now that can be placed by your bedside and will begin to simulate the morning sunrise, slowly getting brighter and brighter to help you wake up. When you awaken sit alongside your light box while you drink your morning tea or coffee or while you read. Within a few days you will begin to notice some nice subtle effects. The light box should be at a 45 degree angle in front of you. Occasionally glance its way as there is no need to stare at it; the full spectrum light passively penetrates your retinas as long as you are looking – reading nearby. It takes most light boxes 30-40 minutes to help balance your serotonin and melatonin levels and its effects will last throughout the day and longer.

Will suntan beds help?

Sun tan beds are not the most effective for helping people with SAD because you have to wear protective eyewear during your tanning session, thereby preventing the bright light from penetrating your retina. Sun booths do emit UVB light which produces vitamin D in the skin, but they also emit UVA light – the light which causes skin aging.

One thing that sun tan beds do which help people suffering with SAD and depression is they stimulate the skin into making beta-endorphins, the feel good chemical that was once thought to only be produced in the brain. Dr. Holick and his colleagues have proven that these beta-endorphins are also produced by exposure to UVB radiation. So, not only will your vitamin D levels increase from UVB radiation from the sun or a sun tanning booth, you will also increase the beta-endorphins coursing through your blood.

Relying on a suntan booth alone however, will not be enough to help with SAD symptoms. It is a good way to augment other light therapies and raise your vitamin D levels at the same time. And remember, like precautions for sun use, avoid overexposure and sunburns. Overuse of the sun booth will damage the skin and increase the risk of skin cancer. There is also the expense to consider.

What's a sun sauna?

Sun Saunas are 'dry' infrared heat saunas with full spectrum lights and are ideal for people experiencing Seasonal Affective Disorder. The dual feature of receiving full spectrum light to balance out brain hormones and also feel like you are being warmed by the sun is a great aid for people with SAD. My patients commonly remark at how their mental attitudes and energy levels soar after their sun sauna visit.

Sun saunas also help your body detox. The infrared heat penetrates the tissue effectively by heating up the core of the body. As a result, the organs increase their metabolic waste production because of the increased circulation. This enhanced circulation helps to carry out waste and toxin debris from deep inside the body to the outside via the skin, lymph and urinary tract. A study performed on 9/11 firefighters subjected to high levels of toxic chemicals showed to be extremely effective at detoxifying their bodies and helped them heal from the inside out.

Even if you are not 'sick' the infrared heat helps to maintain health by helping your body detox more easily. The infrared element is utilized for detoxification from heavy metals and environmental contaminants such as parabens, pthalates and dioxin is remarkable!

So, why not detox your body and get your serotonin at the same time?! Sun sauna owners are also considering adding a third feature – a UVB element for vitamin D production. This is genius. Soon you'll be able to get your sunlight therapy, detox and vitamin D dose all at the same place and at the same time! When this happens, sun saunas will have a huge advantage over the sun tanning booths!!!

Does exercise really help with SAD?

Cardiovascular exercises, such as running and walking, are great at relieving symptoms of SAD and non-seasonal depression. It works by greatly increasing our 'happy hormones' - namely the endorphins. In addition, by exercising outdoors, even on rainy days, some 'light' will get through the retina which will help to balance the brain hormones and relieve SAD symptoms.

What are the nutritional therapies that help SAD patients?

Vitamin D
Optimal levels of vitamin D (above 60 ng/ml) enhance mood and help alleviate SAD symptoms. Have your physician check your 25(OH)D serum levels to get a baseline and work with your physician to get your levels optimal. If you are unable to get your vitamin D from the sunshine, a good starting dose of oral vitamin D would be 2,000 units/day; preferably with food and in the evening. Oral vitamin D supplements can make you sleepy the same way being in the sun can make you tired. Be sure to have your serum levels checked seasonally as they will change.

Fish Oils (EPA/DHA)
Omega-3 fatty acids found in fish oil, particularly DHA, are needed for normal neurotransmitter production. An optimal dose for SAD and depressed patients is 5,000 mg/day with food.

Thyroid
Have your clinician check your TSH (thyroid stimulating hormone), (T_4) free thyroxin, and your (FT_3) tri-odothyronine levels. All three tests are necessary to ascertain the health of your thyroid. By only running the TSH test (most common test) the whole picture is not available. Your levels should be *optimal* and not at the lower end of the normal ranges. Seek out a holistic practitioner or a different physician if your current doctor doesn't believe these 2 other tests are necessary or tries to convince you otherwise.

B Vitamins
All the B vitamins and especially B-6 are imperative to restoring optimal neurotransmitter levels, such as serotonin. A B-complex which is high in B-6 is recommended. A good one that I give my patients is made by Thorne Research - B complex #6. Which ever supplement you choose, your optimal daily intake of B-6 should be 200 mg.

St. John's Wort
St. John's Wort can be helpful in alleviating symptoms of SAD, such as sadness and irritability. It may also help other symptoms such as hopelessness and poor sleep. St. John's Wort is mild and is not recommended for severe depression. It should be taken alone and not with other antidepressants.

Recommended dose: 1,200 – 1,500 mg/day

Contraindications:

- Not recommended for severe depression
- Do not use if you are taking an antidepressant
- Do not combined with 5-HT

5-HT (5-hydroxytryptophan)

5-HT is an amino acid precursor, one step beyond L-tryptophan, in producing serotonin. It is highly effective for treating SAD, especially when there are combined symptoms of insomnia and carbohydrate cravings. It should not be combined with St. John's Wort or any other antidepressant. A good starting dose is 50-100 mg 1 hour before bed. It is highly recommended that you seek out a healthcare professional who can help you with this amino acid and other nutritional therapies.

Starting dose: 50-100 mg 1 hour before bed

Contraindications:

- Do not use if you are taking an antidepressant
- Do not combined with St. John's Wort

Part II: Naturopathic therapies for diseases and conditions linked to vitamin D deficiency

Disclaimer: The following therapies, recommendations and suggestions are in no way intended to treat the diseases and conditions addressed in this book. They are meant to be adjunctive support for consideration under the guidance of your licensed physician.

Chapter 10: Auto-Immune Diseases

Auto-immune diseases are disorders in which your body has been informed by your immune system to attack itself. This can happen for different reasons. One way is for an undigested protein or toxic substance, commonly from the digestive tract, to penetrate the gut wall and enter into the bloodstream where it does not belong. Our antibodies capture this foreign invader and join with it to become an immune complex (IC). It then finds a tissue in the body for which it has an affinity. The immune system (other white blood cells) is alerted to attack and destroy this complex unbeknownst to the tissue it has landed on. Auto immunity can occur in several tissues.

Rheumatoid arthritis: this immune complex (IC) destroys synovial membranes (joints).

Sjogren's syndrome: the (IC) destroys the lacrimal tissues that produce tears and salivary glands (saliva).

Systemic Lupus Erythrematosus (SLE): the IC can destroy several different connective tissues producing pain, stiffness and even kidney damage.

Another less known autoimmune syndrome is Hashimoto's thyroiditis where the IC destroys the thyroid's ability to produce thyroxin.

At this point, most of the focus on autoimmunity has been placed on treating them with pharmaceuticals. Rarely, does the underlying cause of these illnesses get addressed.

The Connection with Vitamin D

There is undisputed proof in the literature demonstrating vitamin D's ability to halt autoimmunity. Since the strong association between optimal D levels and halting the autoimmunity process has been established, correction of reduced or deficient serum levels is a must for everyone!

The serum level that has been shown to control the inflammatory process and shows an alleviation of autoimmunity is 60ng/mL or higher. It is important to determine your baseline 25(OH)D level and work with your practitioner to get it to an optimal level above 60 ng/mL. Be sure your physician is familiar with 'how to dose' for optimal levels. As a highly experienced vitamin D physician, I commonly will prescribe 50,000 units once weekly for 4-8 weeks. I'll recheck levels every 6-8 weeks until they are 65ng/ml or higher and then place them on a maintenance dose.

Other factors to take into account

Food allergens:

Food allergens can precipitate an autoimmune reaction. They play a big role because of the inflammatory upset they cause at the level of the intestinal membrane. This membrane becomes 'leaky' as a result of the undigested food allergens and an open invitation for any toxic substance to enter. This leaky gut must be repaired. By visiting your naturopathic doctor you will get proper guidance on how to correct a leaky gut.

Natural Therapies

Vitamin D
Work with your physician to get your vitamin D serum levels above 60ng/ml.

Fish Oils
EPA/DHA from fish oils act as anti-inflammatory agents. They have a strong affinity for reducing inflammatory reactions in the joints. Since autoimmunity is precipitated by inflammation, incorporating it into your daily regime is wise prevention.

For active inflammation (pain and swelling) add 5,000-6,000 mg to your daily diet.

For mild inflammation add 4,000-5,000 mg/day

Pancreatic enzymes
Pancreatic enzymes (not plant enzymes) are strong therapeutic anti-inflammatory agents. They are highly proteolytic and therefore break-down and digest those nasty blood stream immune complexes (IC's).

Recommended dose: 2 tablets 3 times daily away from food (30-60 minutes before eating).

CMO (Cetyl Myristoleate)
CMO is a joint lubricant and anti-inflammatory agent.

Recommended dose: 540 mg/day.

Lifestyle and Dietary Suggestions

Review with your health care practitioner your food allergens and intolerances to create a healthful diet.

BE PROACTIVE

Maintain your vitamin D levels at or above 60ng/ml.

Find out which food allergens may be causing you a leaky gut and eliminate them.

Eat an anti-inflammatory diet; devoid of cow's milk, red meat, trans-fats, sugars and certain grains.

Include fresh fish, greens, olive, coconut and fish oils.

Chapter 11: Diabetes Type I

Diabetes type I, also known as juvenile diabetes and insulin dependent diabetes. It is a disease in which the beta cells in the islets of the pancreas are destroyed by the immune system. It is not known what caused the immune system to attack itself and destroy these cells, but by the time of diagnosis, it is estimated that 80% of the cells have been destroyed.

The main purpose of the pancreas is to produce insulin; a critical component in the body whose purpose is to take sugar from the blood and move it into the cells of the body to be used as energy.

Insulin is analogous to the gas pump at the gas station. You may be able to pay for the gas, but standing right next to the tank won't make your car run. You need a device that will move the fuel from the underground storage tank to your gas tank. Only a car with gas in its tank will run and only when you have sufficient insulin can your body function properly.

The auto-immune destruction of the insulin producing cells in the pancreas most often targets children and young adults. If a child or young teen lacks sufficient vitamin D levels to protect and support their body, they become at risk for a number of diseases, including diabetes type 1.

Diabetes is a serious disease and must be taken so. Before the cause of diabetes was known and a treatment became available, affected children fell prey to the destructive course of the disease, which ended their lives much too early.

Today, diabetes type 1 is a very treatable disease. With the administration of insulin, a healthy diet and exercise, a long life expectancy is the prognosis.

As far as prevention of type I diabetes is concerned, scientific literature has shown that administration of vitamin D resulted in a reduction in the incidence of type 1 diabetes. This is due to the protective effects of vitamin D that support a healthy immune system and reduce inflammation in the body.

Are you at risk for developing Diabetes Type 1?

- Are you a child or young adult (teen) with low vitamin D levels?

Vitamin D's role in the prevention of Diabetes Type 1

A low vitamin D level means that your whole system is at risk and your own personal health habits and genetics play a role in determining how susceptible you are to developing diseases.

Theoretically, optimal vitamin D levels will protect your body from the viruses that attack the pancreas and any corresponding auto-immune process.

Because vitamin D is such a powerful anti-inflammatory and immune system regulator, people with type II diabetes (the non-insulin dependent diabetes) also show an improvement.

BE PROACTIVE

Increase your vitamin D serum levels to 60 ng/ml or higher.

Use the sun wisely. Allow your children to be exposed regularly to sunshine without sunscreen. Apply sunscreen after an appropriate daily dose is achieved (depending on skin tone). **Strictly avoid sunburns!**

Chapter 12: Multiple Sclerosis (MS)

One of the most amazing things I found in the scientific literature pertains to vitamin D's connection to multiple sclerosis. First of all, the geographic distribution of MS is profound. MS is an unknown disease at the equator. What's more, the numbers of people diagnosed with MS rises right along with the increase in latitude. Basically, the further away from the equator you live, the higher your risk for developing the disease.

Secondly, extensive research in the experimental animal model of MS demonstrates a clear halting of the auto-immune process at therapeutic levels of activated vitamin D.

Multiple sclerosis behaves like an autoimmune disease, where the immune system 'attacks' the myelin sheaths surrounding nerves in the spinal cord and brain, thus destroying the nerves ability to transmit impulses. In addition to MS being an auto-immune disease, there is evidence of other underlying causes such as infections, environmental exposure to toxins and genetic susceptibilities.

2.5 million people worldwide have MS. In the US, 400,000 have MS with another 200 diagnosed each week. Those already diagnosed will notice improved symptoms with healthy vitamin D levels and those at risk can greatly improve their chances of avoiding the disease by reaching and maintaining vitamin D levels above 60ng/ml.

Are you at risk for developing Multiple Sclerosis?

- Are you vitamin D deficient?

- Do you live above 40 degrees latitude?

- Is there a family history of MS?

- Have you been exposed to environmental toxins?

- Have you been exposed to mercury?

Vitamin D's role in the prevention of Multiple Sclerosis

Vitamin D acts as both an anti-inflammatory agent and as a direct inhibitor of the autoimmune process.

In an epidemiological study by Dr. Munger in 2004, women with the highest vitamin D intake experienced a 40% reduction in risk of developing multiple sclerosis.

There is also research that shows keeping serum 25(OH)D levels to greater than 60ng/ml makes it almost impossible to have any further autoimmune process occur in the body. It's fantastic news to learn that the autoimmune destruction of the myelin sheath can be halted, however, research has yet to show us how to regenerate the nerves that have already been damaged.

Natural Therapies

Vitamin D

For prevention: 2,000-4,000 daily to prevent the disease.

For positive diagnosis: If you have been diagnosed with MS; work with a physician who can regularly check serum levels and maintain them at the high end of optimum. (suggested greater than 65ng/ml).

Fish oils

6,000 mg of omega 3's daily

Vitamin B12 (methylcobalmin)

1,000-2,000 units daily (sublingual) helps maintain and restore the nervous system. See your doctor to ensure your levels are optimal.

Borage oil or Evening Primrose oil

3 grams/day of GLA helps decrease inflammation

Natural progesterone

Adding natural progesterone to your system has been known to mitigate MS symptoms

Lifestyle and Dietary Suggestions

Dietary fats: Try avoiding saturated fats from animal meats and dairy products. Instead, eat more fish oils, raw nut oils and linoleic acid. Overall, eating more anti-inflammatory fats like fish and olive oil are helpful.

Gluten: some studies show gluten causes a cross reaction with the myelin sheath. Most naturopaths agree that gluten should be completely removed the diet of patients with MS.

Eat organic whole foods (anti-inflammatory in nature is the best call)

BE PROACTIVE

Vitamin D (serum 25(OH)D should be maintained between 65-90ng/ml

B12 serum levels should be optimal (see doctor for optimal evels)

Remove gluten from diet

Eat an anti-inflammatory diet <u>low</u> in sugar!

Chapter 13: Osteomalacia (Adult Rickets)

Osteomalacia is also known as Adult Rickets and like childhood rickets it is induced by a severe vitamin D deficiency. A deficient level of vitamin D can disrupt the bone building process which results in softening of the bone. Over time, bone pain and muscle weakness become persistent. This is especially true of the elderly population who are kept indoors most of the time and exposed to very little if any natural sunlight. Indeed, while deficient levels of vitamin D can manifest in many ways, because it is utilized by the entire body, the development of osteomalacia is a sure sign of significantly low vitamin D levels.

Osteomalacia vs. Osteoporosis? What's the difference? While both are bone disorders and linked to vitamin D deficiency, and while both can result in bone breakage, the defining difference noticed by patients is the symptoms. Osteomalacia patients experience bone pain and muscle weakness, whereas osteoporosis is known as the silent thief because the diagnosis usually preceeds a bone break because there are no noticeable symptoms beforehand.

On the bright side, even moderate levels of 25(OH)D control inflammation extremely well, and patients with osteomalacia respond well once their blood levels of 25(OH)D have increased to a healthy level (above 60ng/ml).

Are you at risk of developing Osteomalacia?

- Are you vitamin D deficient?

Vitamin D's role in the prevention and treatment of Osteomalacia

Vitamin D acts to decrease inflammatory hormones in the body such as cytokines and interleukins, thereby reducing any boney inflammation.

Vitamin D increases the absorption of calcium which strengthens the bone and alleviates the symptoms.

If increasing vitamin D levels do not ameliorate these symptoms, then consider thyroid issues, arthritis, menopause, fibromyalgia and/or systemic Candida.

Natural Therapies

Vitamin D

A baseline should be established and targeted to 60 ng/ml or higher. Recheck regularly to keep levels on the higher side.

Calcium

Helps to maintain the boney matrix and alkalinize the blood. It also helps vitamin D to work more effectively.

Suggested dose: 1,000 mg of calcium citrate. Take with vitamin D supplement and with food. Avoid taking magnesium with the same meal.

Fish Oils (EPA/DHA)

Reduces inflammation. Suggested dose: 5,000 mg/day.

Boron

Boron stimulates the bony matrix and helps activate vitamin D. Suggested dose: 3 mg/day.

Lifestyle and Dietary Suggestions

Have your serum levels of vitamin D checked by your physician.

BE PROACTIVE

Maintain vitamin D levels over 60 ng/ml.

Help raise your vitamin D levels by exposing your skin to the sun 30 minutes each day (longer if your skin is darker).

Keep inflammation down by eating lots of cold water fish or ingesting 5,000 mg of omega-3 fatty acids daily.

Add a Boron supplement to your diet.

Chapter 14: Osteoporosis

Osteoporosis is called *The Silent Thief*. It's a disease that progresses pain-lessly and without signs or symptoms. Consequently, a diagnosis with osteoporosis usually comes after a bone breaks. Most often the bones that break are the wrist, ribs, spine, hips and legs. These bones break rel-atively easily due to a significant bone loss that developed over time.

Osteoporosis is a disease marked by reduced bone density. It occurs com-monly in women that are post-menopausal or from premature ovarian failure (absence of reproductive hormones, namely estrogen).

Are you at risk of developing Osteoporosis?

- Are you vitamin D deficient?
- Are you fair skinned and thin?
- Are you post-menopausal?
- Are you young and have premature ovarian failure?
- Do you have a sedentary lifestyle?
- Do you have a lack of estrogen?
- Do you have poor mineral absorption?
- Do you have limited exposure to sunlight?
- Do you have poor calcium intake?

Vitamin D's role in the prevention of Osteoporosis

Activated vitamin D and its metabolites are established regulators of bone mineralization and thus play a critical role in maintaining healthy bones.

Natural Therapies

Vitamin D

Establish a baseline before dosing. An optimal level should be attained and maintained. A 25(OH)D serum level over 65 ng/ml is suggested, but have your physician take into account other risk factors.

Calcium Citrate

Helps improve bone density in peri-menopausal women and slows the rate of bone loss in post-menopausal women by 30-50%. Calcium together with vitamin D helps to reduce the risk of hip fractures. Suggested dose: 1,000-1,200 mg/day.

Magnesium

Magnesium helps by normalizing the secretion of parathyroid hormone and calcitonin, which both help to maintain proper calcium concentration in the blood.

Suggested dose: 500 mg/day. **Do not take with vitamin D.**

Boron

Boron helps to activate vitamin D and estrogens, thereby reducing the risk of osteoporosis.

Suggested dose: 3 mg/day.

Other Therapies to consider

Bioidentical hormones

Have your highly experienced anti aging physician ascertain your levels and then optimize them.

If homocysteine levels are high it can interfere with collagen cross-linking which can lead to a defective boney matrix and therefore, osteoporosis. Consider supplementing with B6, B12 and folic acid.

Lifestyle and Dietary Suggestions

There are a number of lifestyle and dietary changes your can make in your life that will positively influence the prevention and/or treatment of osteoporosis.

Establish an exercise routine that includes weight bearing exercises.

Avoid drinking soft drinks because they act to de-mineralize bones.

Limit your alcohol consumption.

Limit your coffee to 2 cups or less per day.

Get outside and enjoy the sunshine.

Take a vitamin D supplement.

Eat a diet high in whole foods and plenty of protein.

Add foods to your diet that are high in calcium such as greens and dairy products.

BE PROACTIVE

Attain and maintain optimal vitamin D levels above 65ng/ml.

Do weight bearing exercises 3-5 days per week

Avoid soft drinks

Limit alcohol and caffeine

Stop smoking

Eat plenty of vegetables, fruits and proteins

Have your bone density checked if you are over 45 or if you have had a fracture as an adult.

Chapter 15: Breast Cancer

Breast cancer, and cancer in general, is characterized by the unregulated replication of cells. This occurs when cells divide improperly or incompletely. They become abnormal and they begin to grow at exponential rates. When this occurs, malignant tumors develop and cancer becomes the diagnosis.

Each year approximately 180,000 women in the United States are diagnosed with breast cancer and another 50,000 women die from this disease. Decades of solid scientific research have shown us that with moderate sun exposure and optimal vitamin D levels, the number of women affected by breast cancer would plummet. Are you wondering how big of an impact the sun and vitamin D supplementation would have if given the chance? **If all women in the US had optimal vitamin D status, there would be 150,000 fewer cases diagnosed each year, and up to 37,000 fewer deaths from breast cancer alone.**

Are you at risk for developing breast cancer?
- Are you vitamin D deficient?
- Are you significantly overweight?
- Do you drink alcohol?
- Did you begin nursing your 1st child after you were 26?
- Were you older than 55 at the time of your last menstrual cycle?

Vitamin D's role in the prevention of Breast Cancer

One of the amazing characteristics of vitamin D, is its ability to perform cellular differentiation, that is, it is able to discern a normal cell from an abnormal cell. When an abnormal cell is identified it is 'taken care of' by the body (targeted for elimination), thereby preventing abnormal cellular growth and tumors. As you can see, having optimal levels of vitamin D in your system goes a long way toward preventing cancer.

Natural Therapies

If you have been diagnosed with breast cancer, consider complimenting your allopathic oncology care with naturopathic medicine. This powerful combination helps patient survival rates and greatly increases your quality of life.

Vitamin D

Prevention: For Breast Cancer prevention your vitamin D levels need to be optimal, which means maintaining levels over 65 ng/ml.

Treatment: If you have been diagnosed with Breast Cancer your optimal serum levels of vitamin D need to be approximately 100 ng/ml.

Preventing Recurrence: To help stay in remission please keep your vitamin D serum levels between 80-90 ng/ml.

Green Tea

Green tea consumption is associated with increased survival time and decreased spread to the lymph glands.

DIM (Diindolymethane)

DIM is a metabolite of indole-3-carbinol (from brassica foods like cabbage and broccoli) which has a positive effect on the metabolism of estrogen into weaker (safer) end products. Dim has also been shown to stimulate the destruction of breast cancer cells. Suggested dose: 100-400 mg/day.

Iodoral

This strong form of organic/inorganic iodine is associated with healthier breast tissue. Suggested dose: 25-50mg/day.

Melatonin

Second after vitamin D, melatonin is the strongest immune surveillance hormone produced by your body. By escalating your dose slowly to 20 mg before bed nightly, you are providing your body with a powerful therapeutic anticancer agent.

CoQ10

For breast cancer prevention: 100-200 mg/day. If positive diagnosis, studies show 390 mg/day is the appropriate dosage to inhibit the spread of cancer (metastasis).

Lifestyle and dietary suggestions

Avoid Daily Consumption of Alcohol. Recent studies show that one drink per day can increase your risk of breast cancer by 10%. Two drinks per day increase risk by 25% and 3-4 drinks per day by 40%. Why? The liver's main job is to break down toxins that are ingested or absorbed into the body. When the liver's detoxification pathway is occupied with regular drinking, the estrogen levels buildup which can cause unchecked cellular replication, otherwise known as cancer.

Folic Acid and Alcohol: There have been studies which show that if women drink and take folic acid it reduces their risk of developing breast cancer, when compared to women who drink and don't take folic acid.

Avoid Sugar. It's long been known that glucose feeds cancer cells. It follows that foods containing sugar can and will increase your risk of developing cancer, including breast cancer. If you have already been diagnosed with cancer, it's advisable to strictly reduce the amount of sugar in your diet.

Sugar also inhibits the immune system by destroying white blood cells.

Eat More Fiber. Consume a diet high in insoluble fibers such as whole grains, psyllium husks and fiber pectins. These types of fibers reportedly lower estrogen levels by binding them in the gut and not allowing the estrogen to recycle back into the bloodstream.

Reduce Consumption of Fats. High fat diets have been shown to increase the risk of developing breast cancer: When women are placed on low fat diets, especially low in meat and dairy fats, their estrogen levels and body fat drop.

BE PROACTIVE

Maintain optimal vitamin D levels

-for prevention: greater than 65 ng/ml

-for active breast cancer: close to 100 ng/ml

-to stay in remission: 80-90 ng/ml

Keep alcohol consumption to a minimum

Keep body fat down by exercising and eating a low fat, low sugar diet

Eat a variety of fibers daily

Chapter 16: Colon Cancer

Colon cancer, also referred to as colorectal cancer, is the second most deadly cancer. The good news is, it is highly curable, especially if detected and treated early.

Are you at risk for developing Colon Cancer?

- Are you vitamin D deficient?
- Do you smoke?
- Do you drink alcohol heavily?
- Are you obese?
- Do you eat a diet high in fat with a high consumption of red meat?
- Are you sedentary and lack exercise in your life?
- Is there a strong family history of colonic polyps, ulcerative colitis and/or Crohn's disease?
- Do you have inflammation in your body?

Vitamin D's role in prevention of Colon Cancer

Vitamin D is anti-carcinogenic and keeps all abnormal cellular proliferation in check. Optimal levels of 25(OH)D in the bloodstream regularly check all abnormal cellular division. When serum 25(OH)D levels are over 40ng/ml the immune surveillance for cancer cells is greatly enhanced. Activated D also encourages cellular apoptosis (cellular suicide for aberrant cells such as cancer) *In other words, vitamin D creates an environment so inhospitable for cancer cells that they'd prefer to kill themselves than continue proliferating.*

Vitamin D also downgrades the inflammatory response and should always be recommended for prevention of colon cancer, since inflammation is directly tied to colon cancer.

How great is your risk of colon cancer with deficient vitamin D levels in your body? Dr. Holick, the leading expert on vitamin D wrote that the research participants in the Women's Health Initiative who began with 25(OH)D levels which were deficient (at or below 12 ng/ml) had a 253%

increase in their risk for colorectal cancer over the next 8 year follow-up period!

Conversely, occupations with the highest exposure to sunlight, and consequently higher vitamin D levels, are associated with significantly reduced death rates from colon cancer.

Natural Therapies

Vitamin D

Prevention: Have your physician check you baseline vitamin D serum levels and maintain at 65—80ng/ml.

As concurrent treatment for cancer diagnosis: 10,000+ IU daily. It's extremely important to obtain a baseline of 25(OH)D and monitor levels every 4-8 weeks when this amount is prescribed. Your holistic physician should be monitoring your blood levels regularly. Again, DO NOT SELF MEDICATE!

Omega-3 fatty acids

EPA and DHA are abundant in cold water fish and they induce apoptosis of colon cancer cells. Suggested dose: 6,000 mg/day.

Melatonin

In cellular studies, melatonin induced apoptosis (cellular death) of human colon cancer cells. It also displayed a direct anti-tumor immune response.

Curcumin

This strong phyto-chemical inhibits cell growth, reduces inflammation and displays apoptosis.

Aged garlic extract

A recent cellular study showed that aged garlic extract has potential to suppress tumor formation and inhibits angiogenesis of colorectal cells.

Resveratrol

Recent studies show that Resveratrol can inhibit colon cancer development.

Flax seed

Flax seed decreases levels of inflammatory cox-1 and cox-2 (inflammatory hormones) and has been shown to help prevent colon cancer development.

<u>Vitamin E Succinate</u>

This form of vitamin E has been shown to inhibit colon cancer cells. It appears to suppress tumor growth through apoptosis and reduces cell proliferation. Suggested dose: 400-800 units/day.

Lifestyle and Dietary Suggestions

Having a healthy lifestyle will reduce your risk of developing cancers in general. A healthy diet and lifestyle does this by giving your body the tools it needs to heal itself. Please note: There are specific dietary restrictions for patients already diagnosed with colon conditions such as ulcerative colitis. Please follow the guidance of your physician. In general, for a healthy colon, follow these suggestions:

Eat a diet rich in fiber.

Find an exercise that you enjoy and make it a regular part of your life.

Eat a diet full of fresh fruits and vegetables.

Reduce consumption of red meat and high fat in your diet.

Keep alcohol consumption to a minimum or eliminate altogether.

Quit smoking (or don't start).

BE PROACTIVE

Maintain vitamin D serum level between 65-80 ng/ml

Maintain optimal serum vitamin D levels to reduce the inflammatory response in the colon, which in turn reduces your risk of colon cancer

Eat a low fat diet

Eat lots of fibers

Exercise regularly

Do not smoke.

Keep alcohol consumption to a minimum

Reduce consumption of red meat

Chapter 17: Lung Cancer

While lung cancer is only the third most commonly diagnosed cancer it is the number one cancer killer. There are two main types or varieties of lung cancer: non-small-cell lung cancer (NSCLC) and small-cell lung cancer (oat-cell lung cancer). Of all lung cancers, 80% fall under the category of non-small-cell lung cancers (NSCLC). These include squamous-cell lung cancer, adenocarcinoma, and large cell carcinoma. Small-cell lung cancers are much less common and are more invasive.

Are you at risk for developing Lung Cancer?

- Are you a smoker? The American Lung Association reports that 87% of lung cancers are caused by smoking tobacco products and second hand exposure.

- Have you been or do you regularly expose yourself to secondhand smoke?

- Are you or have your been exposed to radon gas? Radon gas exposure is the 2nd leading cause of lung cancer.

- Are you exposed to workplace carcinogens such as asbestos, arsenic, uranium and/or air pollutants? These pollutants are also known to cause lung cancer.

- Are you vitamin D deficient? Vitamin D deficiency directly increases risk of developing lung cancer.

Vitamin D's role in prevention of Lung Cancer

There has been significant research done at University of California, San Diego on the role of vitamin D and lung cancer. What they've found is an inverse relationship between sunlight exposure and lung cancer, with the sunlight exposure determined by latitude. The study showed that lung cancer rates were lowest near the equator (most sunlight) and steadily rose the further away people were from the equator (least sunlight). This is further evidence of the powerful effects of activated vitamin D and its strong anti-carcinogenic characteristics.

Additionally, researchers have shown that smokers who have a protective level of vitamin D have a much higher rate of surviving lung cancer compared with patients living in areas of the country where low vitamin D levels are prevalent due to the latitude and climate. In a study by Dr. Hyun-Sook Lim et.al., <u>Cancer Survival is dependent on season of diagnosis and sunlight exposure,</u> he writes, "We also found sunlight exposure to be a predictor of cancer survival."

And as vitamin D acts to modulate inflammation in the body, the effects on a cellular level is to correct precancerous cells by way of apoptosis (death).

Natural Therapies

Vitamin D

Prevention: 2,000-4,000 units/day until levels reach greater than 70 ng/ml

Treatment for lung cancer patients: Vitamin D levels should be maintained at greater than 80ng/ml.

Antioxidants

Yale University found a strong correlation between dietary antioxidant intake and reduced lung cancer in male smokers.

Carotenoids, vitamin C, vitamin E, selenium, flavinoids are all beneficial antioxidants.

Curcumin

This herbal anti-inflammatory has been shown to induce apoptosis in human non-small–cell lung cancer in vitro.

Melatonin

A very strong antioxidant exerts anti-cancer effects in vitro. There is a study that shows that both the overall tumor regression rate and survival rate were much higher in patients who were treated with melatonin along with chemotherapy.

Fish Oils

Omega-3 fatty acids EPA and DHA are anti-inflammatory and have been shown (EPA) to inhibit growth of lung cancer cells in vitro.

Lifestyle and dietary suggestions

The most effective way to build your health and ward off risk of lung cancer is to eliminate your exposure to the toxins that have been linked to causing lung cancer. It also doesn't matter how long your exposure has been: by removing the toxins now, you will activate your body's natural healing processes. Avoid exposure to radon gas, workplace carcinogens, secondhand smoke and most importantly, if you are a smoker, take steps to stop today. If you've tried to stop smoking and started again, give yourself a pat on the back. For whatever period of time you were not smoking, you were helping your body. Now, do it again. Quit smoking as many times as you have to until you stay that way. Remember, if you really want to stop, you can. There are plenty of helpful resources to move you from a smoker to a non-smoker, and being a non-smoker is the best way to reduce your risk of lung cancer.

BE PROACTIVE

Cessation of smoking and exposure to second hand smoke are essential steps to decreasing your risk of lung cancer.

Maintain optimal vitamin D serum levels

For prevention: greater than 70 ng/ml

For lung cancer patients: 80-100 ng/ml

Avoid environmental toxins such as radon gas, asbestos, uranium, arsenic and air pollutants.

Avoid environmental estrogens such as pesticides and insecticides.

Eat lots of fruit and vegetables, organic when possible.

Add a green tea supplement in addition to drinking green tea to induce apoptosis of lung cancer cells.

Chapter 18: Pancreatic Cancer

The pancreas is the gland in our abdomen responsible for producing insulin, hormones and digestive enzymes. Pancreatic cancer is the fourth leading cause of cancer in the U.S. Although it is less common, once diagnosed it can have a poor prognosis since metastasis may occur quickly.

Are you at risk for developing Pancreatic Cancer?

- Are you a smoker?
- Do you have diabetes?
- Do you have a larger waist to hip circumference?
- Do you eat a diet high in fat content?
- Do you or have you had exposure to carcinogens?
- Are you vitamin D deficient?

Vitamin D's role in the prevention of Pancreatic Cancer

Vitamin D deficiency has shown to make a person much more susceptible to pancreatic cancer. Its probable role is that of a strong anti-inflammatory agent to the pancreatic tissue.

Natural Therapies

Vitamin D

Maintain your serum levels between 65-85 ng/ml for protective prevention.

If already diagnosed, have your physician monitor your levels regularly and maintain them between 80 and 100 ng/ml.

Green tea

The active compound found in green tea, EGCG, may reduce proliferation and invasion of pancreatic cancer cells.

Omega 3 fatty acids

EPA and DHA have both been shown to inhibit pancreatic cancer cell growth. DHA, in particular can induce pancreatic cellular apoptosis.

Alpha-lipoic acid

A very strong anti-oxidant which helps to induce apoptosis and reduce inflammation. Intravenous alpha-lipoic acid has been used with some success for patients with metastasized pancreatic cancer.

Folic Acid

One study has shown that increased dietary intake of folic acid (folate) was associated with a reduced risk.

Pancreatin

Pancreatic enzymes have been used for decades for digestion. By ingesting them on an empty stomach these powerful proteolytic enzymes can breakdown and digest cancer cells, bacteria, viruses, etc.

Curcumin

Can suppress the growth of human pancreatic cancer cells as well as stimulate 'cell death' (apoptosis).

Protein intake

The protein intake of patients diagnosed with pancreatic cancer needs to be higher. I recommend 60-100 grams daily of healthy protein along with pancreatic enzymes as crucial to help maintain muscle mass and cellular nutrition.

Lifestyle and Dietary Suggestions

Diets that are high in fat and cholesterol significantly increase the risk of pancreatic cancer. Another recent study taken from the International Journal of Cancer confirmed that red meat intake increased the risk of pancreatic cancer.

Having a larger waist circumference that hip circumference also may predict insulin resistance and is also a risk factor.

A sedentary lifestyle may also contribute.

A diet high in cruciferous vegetables may also reduce your risk of pancreatic cancer.

BE PROACTIVE

Maintain optimal vitamin D levels.

<u>For prevention</u>: maintain levels between 65-85 ng/ml.

<u>For pancreatic cancer patients</u>: maintain levels of 80 ng/ml or higher.

Stop smoking.

Stop drinking alcohol.

If you are overweight or obese, work with your physician to reduce your body fat. Keeping a healthy body mass index, you will reduce your risk for pancreatic cancer in addition to feeling better and having more energy.

Exercise regularly.

Keep fats and red meat to a minimum.

Omega-3 fatty acids, alpha-lipoic acid and folic acid are just a few vital supplements which help to prevent and/or fight pancreatic cancer.

Have your physician monitor your baseline vitamin D levels and re-check every 2-3 months, and especially when the seasons change.

Chapter 19: Prostate Cancer

Prostate cancer is the most commonly diagnosed cancer. It begins in the glandular cells of the prostate and is known as adenocarcinoma. When prostate cancer is diagnosed early and confined to the prostate a long term disease free survival is often the prognosis. If the cancer has advanced but is contained locally, the prognosis is good and long term survival is also likely. In the unfortunate case that the cancer has metastasized to distant organs, the prognosis may be only one to three years life expectancy.

Prostate cancer, like all cancers, is characterized by unregulated replication of cellular growth resulting in tumors. Prostate cancer is a very common cancer in men in the U.S. and typically develops after 40. It has commonly been associated with hormonal imbalances.

Are you at risk for developing Prostate Cancer?

- Are you male?   Prostate cancer is a strictly male disease because only men have a prostate gland.

- Do you have a dark skin tone? African American men have the highest incidence of prostate cancer. They also have a tendency toward being more vitamin D deficient.

- Are you vitamin D deficient?

- Are you over 40?

- Do you eat a diet high in red meats and dairy products and low in fruits and vegetables?

- Do you have a sedentary lifestyle?

- Do you have a family history of prostate cancer? If your father or brother was diagnosed with prostate cancer, your risk of developing prostate cancer is doubled.

Vitamin D's role in the prevention of Prostate Cancer

Vitamin D plays a significant role in prostate cancer prevention. Several studies have demonstrated that vitamin D can inhibit prostate cancer growth. The research is laden with studies that more than prove the disarming of prostate cancer cells with vitamin D supplementation. Vitamin

D keeps abnormal cells like cancer in check and allows apoptosis (cellular death) to occur to these cells. Vitamin D is also anti-proliferative, and as such makes it difficult for cancer cells to grow.

The prostate gland is one of the unique organs in the body that can activate it's own vitamin D. Vitamin D also acts as a strong inhibitor of inflammation and plays the role of director of cell regulation and replication. Unfortunately, if vitamin D is missing from your internal 'mileau' you have no director and cells will be allowed to run amuck causing unregulated abnormal cell growth, also known as cancer. Activated vitamin D in optimal levels in the body is the most powerful nutrient to protect against prostate cancer.

Natural Therapies

Vitamin D

Prevention: 2,000-10,000 units/day depending on your baseline levels of serum 25(OH)D. An optimal level of 75-85 ng/ml will be very protective. Have your physician monitor your blood levels as your levels rise quickly with a higher dose. Check serum levels every 3-6 months till you reach an optimal level. Once you reach an optimum level, discuss with your physician how to maintain this level safely.

Treatment: Maintain serum vitamin D levels between 80-100 ng/ml.

DIM (diindole methane)

200-400 mg/day for treatment

Lycopene

30-50 mg/day for prevention

Carotenoid complex

A very strong anticancer antioxidant. 25,000 – 50,000 units/day with food for prevention.

CoQ10

100 mg/day may help lower human prostate cancer cell growth.

Curcumin

Has been shown to help prevent prostate cancer by lowering inflammatory hormone levels.

Green tea

A potent agent against prostate cancer.

Melatonin

Up to 20 mg at night may inhibit growth of cancer cells.

Omega-3 fatty acids

A dosage of approximately 1,000 mg/day of EPA (eicosapentaenoic acid) prevents apoptosis and decreases proliferation of prostate cancer cells.

Modified citrus pectin

This derivative of citrus helps in preventing metastasis of the prostate cancer; thereby slowing down the spread and growth of cancer.

Lifestyle and Dietary Suggestions

Avoidance of Alcohol: There is an association with prostate cancer and alcohol consumption. This is likely due to the liver detoxification pathways being occupied with alcohol and unavailable for processing testosterone.

In general, avoid over consumption of meat products.

Flax, canola and soy oils maybe helpful.

Eat lots of cruciferous vegetables such as cabbage, broccoli and brussel sprouts. Anything in the "fica" family of veggies shows anticancer activity.

BE PROACTIVE

Maintain optimal vitamin D serum level

For prevention: greater than 65 ng/ml

For prostate cancer patients: 80-100 ng/ml

Eat lots of cruciferous vegetables daily.

Eat lots of greens and fibers daily.

Avoid red meat and too much dairy.

Avoid alcohol.

Have a PSA (Prostate Specific Antigen) tests done yearly.

Other helpful nutrients which help prostate cancer are: omega 3-fatty acids, modified citrus pectin and melatonin.

Chapter 20: Ovarian Cancer

"In general, ovarian cancer incidence and mortality is higher
in northern than southern latitudes... Conclusion: this
ecologic study supports the hypothesis that sunlight may be
a protective factor for ovarian cancer mortality."
*Lefkowitz, E.S. and Garland, C.F. Sunlight, vitamin D, and
ovarian cancer mortality rates in US women.*

The ovaries are key endocrine glands of the female reproductive system
and several types of tumors can form in the ovaries. Approximately 5-10%
of ovarian cancers are familial (genetic predisposition). These cancers are
usually associated with inherited mutations of BRCA1 and BRCA2 genes.

In 2005, 16,000 women died from ovarian cancer in the same year they
were diagnosed (out of 22,000 total diagnosed). Prognosis does appear to
be more favorable in women diagnosed at a younger age with a lower
stage of the disease and good performance status at diagnosis (able to
function normally).

Unfortunately, many women are not 'caught' in the early stages of the
cancer due to its difficulty to diagnose initially. Since in its earlier stages,
ovarian cancer presents few symptoms. As it progresses symptoms can
include abdominal pain or cramps, pain in the lower back and pelvis,
abnormal vaginal bleeding, bloating, enlargement of the belly and so on.

Are you at risk for developing Ovarian Cancer?

- Do you have a family history of ovarian cancer?

- Are you vitamin D deficient?

- Have you previously had breast cancer?

- Were you unable to have children due to infertility?

- Have you given birth? (If you answered no, your risk is higher)

Vitamin D's role in the prevention of Ovarian Cancer

Activated vitamin D acts as an anti-inflammatory and apoptotic agent to
the ovarian tissue. Since the ovaries are one of the unique tissues that can
activate its own vitamin D they are more vulnerable to cancer without a

sufficient amount. Activated vitamin D has shown to significantly inhibit the growth of ovarian cancer cells. The receptor sites for vitamin D on the ovaries (VDR's) when occupied with activated vitamin D act to inhibit growth signaling pathways, thereby controlling any unusual cellular growth.

Additionally, there are studies which cite how insufficient vitamin D levels may actually trigger ovarian cancer in a predisposed female.

Natural Therapies

Vitamin D

Prevention: 2,000-4,000 units/day with food is suggested. (This dose should be taken if you are an area of the country where there is a vitamin D winter, or you don't get out in the sun – see chart for optimal D from sunshine) Make certain your levels are maintained at 65 ng/ml or higher.

For ovarian cancer patients: Your healthcare practitioner should guide you with this dosage; make certain they therapeutically dose you initially (treat you at a higher dose until your levels are over 80ng/ml). Maintaining an upper range of 80-100ng/ml may be ideal; this again should be regularly checked every 2-3 months.

Antioxidants

As with any other cancer, vitamins C, E, carotinoid complex, CoQ10 and selenium make great therapeutic agents in cleaning up cellular oxidation and as an adjunct to chemotherapy.

Curcumin

A recent in vitro study demonstrated that curcumin inhibits the growth of ovarian cancer cells.

Green tea

EGCG from green tea has recently demonstrated ovarian cancer cell growth inhibition.

Soy

A recent cellular study has demonstrated that genestein and daidzein from soy reduce ovarian cancer cell proliferation. Soy in the form of fermented soy extract may help with stabilization after chemotherapy for ovarian cancer.

Vitamin A

Vitamin A inhibits the growth of several ovarian tumor cell lines. It helps by blocking the cell cycle progression of ovarian carcinoma cells. It also helps to induce apoptosis (cell differentiation).

Quercitin

This is a strong bio-flavinoid and has been shown to exert a dose-dependent inhibition of ovarian cancer cell growth. It also blocks the tumor's ability to get adequate nutrition.

Lifestyle and Dietary Suggestions

Several studies have demonstrated that there are lifestyle and dietary factors which can prevent ovarian cancer. Exercise has been shown to do this by immune stimulation, hormone balancing and by controlling obesity. Also, women who eat a diet high in vegetables have been shown to have a reduced rate of ovarian cancer. Cow's milk, because of high estrogen content (pregnant cows), has been cited as a potential cause of ovarian cancer. Also, women who drink green and black tea (high in flavinoids) are less likely to develop ovarian cancer.

BE PROACTIVE

Maintain optimal vitamin D serum levels.

For prevention: 65 ng/ml or higher

For ovarian cancer patients: 80-100ng/ml

Seek a medical diagnosis for unexplained vaginal bleeding or abdominal pain

Eat a diet rich with vegetables

Avoid cow's milk

Exercise regularly

Maintain a healthy BMI (Body Mass Index)

Add green and black tea to your diet

Chapter 21: Skin Cancer

Oddly enough, activated vitamin D actually protects the skin from developing skin cancer. In one study direct photo-protective effects of activated vitamin D were observed in skin cells (keratinocytes). Vitamin D protects many cells from oxidative DNA damage, including the skin. For more information on skin cancer and skin health see Chapter 7: Shedding Light on Skin Health and Skin Cancer.

Are you at risk for developing Skin Cancer?

- Did you experience any bad sun burns as a child? This is the one indicator that dramatically increases the risk of developing melanoma.

- Are you vitamin D deficient?

- Are you fair-skinned?

Vitamin D's role in the prevention of Skin Cancer

Vitamin D protects the skin from cancer by way of its anti-inflammatory effect and through cellular differentiation. Vitamin D also acts to activate the skin's immune system.

Natural therapies

Vitamin D

Prevention: 65 ng/ml or higher.

For skin cancer patients: 80-100 ng/ml.

Green Tea

Helps to protect against skin cancer and other cancers.

Carotenioids

Carotenoids are protective for keratinocytes (skin cells). Suggested dose: 25,000-50,000 units/day

Lifestyle and Dietary Suggestions

DO NOT BURN YOUR SKIN. Sunburns predispose you to skin cancer by destroying the cell's immune systems.

When you are in the sun, expose your skin for your minimal erthyemic dose (MED). Your MED will depend on the color of your skin (how much natural protection you have from the sunlight), the time of day and the season. A general estimate would be the amount of time you can stay in the sun BEFORE your skin turns PINK (NOT RED).   After this point, apply sunscreen to your skin to prevent burning and to prevent the destruction of the vitamin D you've just synthesized in your skin.

BE PROACTIVE

DO NOT BURN YOUR SKIN!

Use sunscreen or clothing to protect your skin when you stay outdoors AFTER you've gotten your personal dose of sunlight

Maintain optimal vitamin D levels over 65 ng/ml. Check these levels regularly to ensure you are protected.

Take plenty of green tea and carotenoid rich foods in your diet.

Chapter 22: Cardiovascular: Hypertension

The published research on blood pressure shows a linear rise in blood pressure at increasing distances from the equator. Blood pressures in general also appear to be higher in the winter than in the summer months. Low vitamin D levels from either lack of sun, lack of oral vitamin D supplementation and high skin melanin content are both associated with increased parathyroid hormone secretion and low vitamin D stores. This can cause changes in the vascular smooth muscle and increase its contractibility which can increase blood pressure.

Are you at risk of developing Hypertension?

- Are you vitamin D deficient?

- Is there a family history of hypertension?

- Do you have a dark skin tone?

- Are you overweight?

- Do you use steroids, contraceptive pills, or decongestants?

Vitamin D's role in the prevention and treatment of Hypertension

Vitamin D acts along with the parathyroid and calcium to make vascular changes to smooth muscle controlling blood pressure. Without sufficient vitamin D levels this system is thrown out of balance, which can result in a rise in blood pressure and over time the development of hypertension.

Natural Therapies

Vitamin D

A baseline level of 25(OH)D should be evaluated and treated accordingly. If you have one or more above risk factors, it is a good idea to check levels 3-4 times a year to make sure levels are optimal.

Prevention: 65 ng/ml or higher

For hypertension patients: consult with your physician.

Omega 3 Fatty acids (Flax or Fish oil)

Helps to maintain a healthy blood pressure. Suggested dose: 5,000 mg/day.

Magnesium citrate

Magnesium relaxes the heart muscle and also counters sodium levels, both of which act to lower high blood pressure. Suggested dose: 500-1,000 mg/day.

Garlic

Helps to reduce both the systolic and diastolic blood pressures. Suggested dose: 10 mg/day of allicin.

Coenzyme Q10 (CoQ10)

Lowers blood pressure by stabilizing the vascular system. Suggested dose: 100-300 mg/day.

Potassium

Potassium has been shown to lower both the systolic and diastolic pressures, especially in the elderly and when patients are not responding well to their medications.

Lifestyle and Dietary Suggestions

Maintaining a healthy weight, minimizing alcohol consumption and exercising regularly all help to reduce blood pressure.

BE PROACTIVE

Maintain optimal vitamin D levels over 65 ng/mL

Stop smoking

Exercise regularly

Expose your skin to the sun and/or increase your oral vitamin D if low

Calcium, magnesium and potassium levels are important minerals to maintain at a healthy level

Chapter 23: Immune System Health

Viruses run amuck in the wintertime. This may very well be due in part to the fact that higher levels of vitamin D in our bloodstream are now at a low point. The VDR's in our white blood cells actually help turn on our antiviral defenses. So, if activated D is now low, there is not much artillery for our white blood cells to destroy the enemy viruses.

There are a variety of viruses which can attack and 'take over' the host if vitamin D levels are not optimal. Influenza, the common cold viruses, herpetic viruses, bacteria and fungi are all susceptible to activated vitamin D.

Are you at risk for a compromised Immune System?

- Are you vitamin D deficient?

- Have you been treated for cancer with chemotherapy or radiation?

- Are you run down, stressed or overwhelmed?

- Have you taken lots of antibiotics?

- Do you have poor self-talk, self-esteem or self-image? Studies have shown that your mindset is linked to your immune system. Good healthy thoughts help create a strong immune system.

Vitamin D's role in creating a strong Immune System

Vitamin D activates the natural killer cells for the immune system that act as an army to kill the invading microbial enemies. When the vitamin D receptors on the white blood cells becomes activated the WBC's can perform at their highest level of immune system surveillance.

Natural Therapies

Vitamin D

Prevention: See your physician to monitor your blood levels over 65ng/ml.

For a compromised immune system: 80-100 ng/ml.

Ashwaganda

Lowers chronically elevated cortisol, enhances energy and reduces anxiety.

Astragalus

This herb enhances the cytotoxicity and activity of natural killer cells and macrophages.

Garlic

Enhances natural killer cells function and may increase the tumor cells 'ability' to induce an immune response. Garlic has been shown to inhibit carcinogenesis by helping repair damaged DNA.

Coenzyme Q10 (CoQ10)

Coenzyme Q10 is a potent antioxidant and nutrient that enhances natural killer cell and T cell activity. It is free radical scavenger and prevents cellular damage. CoQ10 also increases cellular production of energy.

Curcumin

Is a strong antioxidant phytochemical. It directly enhances the phagocystic processes of macrophages. It also inhibits tumor growth by blocking the production of inflammatory cytokines.

Echinacea

A popular 'antiviral' botanical which stimulates activity of natural killer cells, macrophages and lymphocytes.

Green Tea

A powerful antioxidant 'camelia sinensis' acts by promoting DNA repair and encourages 'apoptosis' of damaged cells.

Melatonin

An antioxidant hormone that increases the cytotoxic activity of lymphocytes. It is a strong anti-inflammatory and increases T-cell immune activity.

Mushroom polysaccharides

Can stimulate lymphocytes and natural killer cells to secrete cytokines and interferon which can activate a very important path for killing cancer cells.

Vitamin A

Found in fish oils and is an integral part of mucous membrane health. It acts by increasing neutrophils, macrophages and natural killer cells. Vitamin A is required in the development of both helper T and B cells.

Vitamin C

Supports cytotoxic activity and phagocytosis (engulfing bad cells) of lymphocytes and natural killer cells.

Vitamin E

Decreases immune suppression caused by free radicals.

Zinc

A strong anti-oxidant and immuno-stimulant, it helps natural killer cells to destroy virus or cancer cells and helps to produce interleukin-1, an immune regulating protein.

Probiotics

These are 'friendly' bacteria living in the gastrointestinal tract. They aid in nutrient absorption, healthy immune responses and reducing inflammation and infection throughout the body.

Carotenoids

Cofactors for vitamin A production.

Pancreatic enzymes

Proteolytic enzymes from an animal which digest foreign proteins in the blood stream such as antigens, viruses, bacteria, cancer cells, etc....

Lifestyle and Dietary Suggestions

Immune system health can be greatly enhanced by:

Active lifestyle: studies have shown that immunity is enhanced by exercise.

Maintaining a healthy BMI (Body Mass Index) ensures a healthier immune system due to lower body fat. Since body fat approximates a higher insulin level, which impairs the immune system, it is ideal to maintain a healthy weight.

Sugar and refined carbs can destroy our white blood cells, thus contributing to viral activity.

BE PROACTIVE

Maintain optimal vitamin D levels at or above 65 ng/ml

Exercise regularly

Reduce stress in your life

Adopt a healthy outlook and positive self talk

Reach and maintain a healthy BMI

Eat a healthy diet: rich in fruits, vegetable and lower fat proteins

Avoid over consumption of red meats and dairy

Chapter 24: Autism

The Connection between the Brain and Vitamin D

Vitamin D appears to be a crucial neuro-steroid for brain development. Vitamin D receptors are found in most areas of the developing fetal brain which implies its importance for neurodevelopment. It also appears that vitamin D offers neuroprotection; thereby insuring neurotransmitters and hormones interact correctly together which helps in regulating behaviors. Much of this work has been studied by Dr. Alan Kalueff ('06, '07) at the National Institute of Mental Health, where he reviewed the brain enhancing properties of vitamin D. The research stresses the importance of the mother having enough vitamin D while pregnant and the baby acquiring sufficient amounts of vitamin D after birth for normal brain functioning. Vitamin D does this by stimulating a nerve growth factor in the brain of the developing baby.

Activated vitamin D also stimulates neurotrophins, which help nerve cells survive, and increases antioxidant levels of glutathione which reduces metabolic waste products such as calcium and nitrous oxide.

Dr. John McCrath of University of Queensland, Australia, points out that vitamin D deficiency should be examined in more detail as a candidate risk factor for neurodevelopmental disorders.

Production of the VDR in the developing brain increases steadily several weeks after conception. Activated vitamin D via the VDR induces nerve growth factor and stimulates neural (brain cell) growth. Recently, Professor Feron, Dr. Ameras and their group from the University of Marseilles found developmental vitamin D deficiency disrupts 36 proteins involved in brain development. In animal studies they found that severe vitamin D deficiency leads to rat pups with increased brain size and enlarged brain chambers; abnormalities very similar to those found in autistic children.

Not surprisingly, inflammation abnormalities are associated with both Autism and vitamin D deficiency. Autistic people demonstrate proof of chronic inflammation and oxidative stress of both blood and brain.

Is your child at risk for developing Autism?

- Are you pregnant and have a vitamin D deficiency?
- Are you breastfeeding and have a vitamin D deficiency?

- Do you live at a Northern latitude?
- Do you put sunscreen on your child BEFORE they go outside?
- Do you supplement a breast fed or formula fed infant or toddler with vitamin D? If no, there is an increased risk that your child could be vitamin D deficient.
- Is your child vitamin D deficient?

Vitamin D's role in preventing and treating Autism

Vitamin D acts as a potent neural anti-inflammatory to 'quell' the fire in the brain. The inflammatory hormone cascade produced by autistic brains or vitamin D deficient brains can cause severe impairment. Vitamin D helps to decrease the production of inflammatory cytokines in the brain which cause this impairment.

Women who are pregnant, and those who have given birth and are now breast feeding, may believe that they are not vitamin D deficient because they take a prenatal multi-vitamin. The unfortunate reality is that the 400 IU of vitamin D a day is nowhere near sufficient to keep levels optimal. In Dr. Holick's published research, Vitamin D Deficiency, he states that of the women in the study, "70% took a prenatal vitamin, 90% ate fish and 93% drank approximately 2.3 glasses of milk per day, (yet) 73% of the women and 80% of their infants were vitamin D deficient (25-hydroxyvitamin D level, <20ng per milliliter) at the time of birth".

Natural Therapies for Autism

Vitamin D

See a licensed physician who is acquainted with vitamin D's role in autism. Start with a baseline level and work to achieve a more optimal level of 65-80 ng/ml. Recheck this level every 2-3 months. A finger stick blood draw might be easier for a child than a blood draw.

DHA

DHA is derived from fish oil and is a potent omega-3 anti-inflammatory and neural nutrient.

Suggested dose: 600+ mg/day

Folic acid

Suggested dose: 800 mcg/day (5-methyl tetra hydrofolate is the best form)

Vitamin B12

Suggested dose: 1,000+/day (methyl cobalmin – sublingual)

Vitamin C

Suggested dose: 500-1,000 mg/day

B6 or pyridoxal-5-phosphate

Suggested dose: 50-100 mg/day

Magnesium

Suggested dose: 100 mg/day

Lifestyle and Dietary Suggestions

Eliminate wheat and gluten containing foods

Add foods high in sulfur or garlic, legumes, onions and eggs

BE PROACTIVE

Optimize vitamin D levels during pregnancy, especially if not living in a sunny area or if you are not being exposed to sun often.

Continue vitamin D administration to your child postpartum via breast feeding (while mom is taking oral vitamin D) and/or oral drops to baby if drinking formula.

Avoid environmental contaminants such as vaccines containing mercury.

Support healthy fetal development with optimal amounts of fish oil for the DHA content.

Chapter 25: Depression

Depression is a neurotransmitter imbalance in the brain. It can cause fatigue, apathy of different levels, poor motivation, sleep disorders, appetite disorders and poor concentration and focus.

Are you at risk for Depression?

- Are you vitamin D deficient?

- Do you have a family history of depression?

- Are you under significant stress?

- Do you have poor thyroid activity?

- Are you experiencing menopause?

- Do you live above the 35th parallel? Living at a latitude above the 35th parallel puts you at a higher risk for becoming vitamin D deficient due to a 'vitamin D winter'.

Vitamin D's role in the prevention and treatment of depression

Activated vitamin D, via the VDR, increases the genetic expression of tyrosine dydroxylase, which in turn, helps to produce catecholamines/neurotransmitters for brain activity. Since activated vitamin D is so closely tied to the biosynthesis of neurotransmitters, lack of its presence in the brain can cause mild to severe depression.

Interestingly, depression has significant co-morbidity with illnesses associated with low vitamin D levels, such as heart disease, diabetes, osteoporosis, rheumatoid arthritis and hypertension.

Natural Therapies

Vitamin D

Establish a baseline 25(OH)D level through your licensed physician.

Prevention: Optimal levels are between 65-80 ng/ml. Check this level every 2-3 months to maintain this higher level.

For depression patients: 80-100 ng/ml.

Fish oil

(EPA/DHA) Omega 3 fatty acids help decrease neural inflammation and help to balance neurotransmitter activity as well. Suggested dose: 5,000-6,000 mg of omega 3's daily.

For Seasonal Affective Disorder (SAD)

Consider full spectrum light box therapy as outlined in Chapter 9. Suggested dose: 30 minutes in the AM during winter.

5-MTHF

A superior form of folic acid which helps with methylation of homocysteine and is highly effective with neurotransmitter regulation. Suggested dose: 1,000-5,000 mcg/day.

Vitamin B12 – Methylcobalmin

This form of B12 has superior absorption qualities for the nervous system. B12 is a highly effective albeit very neglected nutrient for depression.

5HTP

A potent precursor to serotonin and highly effective for insomnia, carbohydrate cravings and headaches which are all related to low serotonin deficiency. Suggested dose: 50-100 mg (one to three times per day).

Thyroid

Have your physician check your free T3 levels.

Lifestyle and Dietary Suggestions

Participate in a regular cardiovascular exercise program. Exercise reduces stress that can lead to depression. It also releases endorphins which help give you a positive outlook on life.

Limit the amount of caffeine in your drinks. Caffeine gives you an artificial 'high' and then your energy drops.

Eat a healthy and balanced diet full of vegetables and fruit and protein.

Other Mental Health Disorders

While it's certainly understood that most mental health issues do not originate from vitamin D deficiency, having adequate activated levels will have a positive influence on the brains chemistry. Activated vitamin D is, after all, the most powerful hormonal steroid available and achieving optimal levels will be of benefit to any mental health treatment program.

BE PROACTIVE

Attain and maintain optimal vitamin D levels at or above 65 ng/ml.

Optimize B12 levels and folate levels

Expose yourself to full spectrum lighting daily if possible

Exercise (cardiovascular) helps to produce endorphins which are 'feel good' brain hormones

Chapter 26: Skin: Psoriasis

Psoriasis is a skin disease marked by inflammation and marked skin cell turnover. The symptoms of Psoriasis are red flaky skin patches and can be itchy at times.

Are you at risk for developing Psoriasis?

- Do you have a family history of psoriasis?
- Do you have a family history of rheumatoid arthritis?
- Do you have a family history of intestinal dysbiosis (Candida/yeast)?
- Do you have viral or bacterial infections?
- Do you consume alcohol?

Vitamin D's role in the prevention and treatment of Psoriasis

Vitamin D down-regulates inflammations in T-cell cytokines. Vitamin D helps with T-cell differentiation which inhibits pro-inflammatory reactions such as psoriasis.

Natural Therapies

Vitamin D

Establish a baseline with your physician then increase levels over 65 ng/ml. This could also be coupled with a topical vitamin D analogue cream.

Hydrastis

This is a strong botanical which kills fungus in the gut, inhibits undigested proteins into polyamines. Suggested dose: 250-500 mg twice daily. DO NOT TAKE IF PREGNANT.

Fish oils (EPA/DHA)

Fish oils down-regulate inflammation. Suggested dose: 5,000 mg/day.

Zinc picolinate

Adequate levels of zinc are required so that the immune system can heal and inflammation is controlled. Suggested dose: 30 mg/day

Vitamin A

Make sure your physician is on board with you taking this vitamin supplement as it is not a water soluble vitamin and can build up in the tissues over time. DO NOT TAKE WHILE YOU ARE PREGANANT. Suggested dose: 10,000-50,000 units/day.

Lifestyle and Dietary Suggestions

Eat a high fiber diet that includes lots of vegetables, fruit and non-gluten grains. It is equally important to limit the amount of sugar, alcohol, red meat and dairy that you consume in your diet.

BE PROACTIVE

Maintain optimal vitamin D levels at or above 65 ng/ml

Use topical vitamin D as recommended by your physician

Eat lots of fiber including vegetables and fruit and non-gluten grains

Avoid gluten

Limit sugars, alcohol, red meat and dairy in diet

Appendix A: Frequently Asked Questions

What nutrients interact and negate vitamin D?

Vitamin A and magnesium should not be taken within several hours of ingesting oral vitamin D because of their ability to block vitamin D's absorption.

What nutrients/foods help with vitamin D's absorption?

Calcium is one of the most important nutrients that works alongside vitamin D to help increase its effectiveness. Calcium can be taken at the same time as vitamin D, but it can also be taken separately.

Because vitamin D is oil based, eating a meal that contains some oil or fat (i.e. salad dressing or butter) then directly ingesting your oral vitamin D will improve vitamin D's absorption.

How can I find out if I need to be taking vitamin D?

Have your physician test your 25(OH)D levels. This will get you a baseline and inform you and your physician if you need to be getting more sunshine, or be taking an oral vitamin D supplement.

How can I raise my vitamin D levels?

If you live in a sunny area, you have the opportunity to get your vitamin D from the sunshine by going outside often. Remember to put sunscreen on after you've gotten your daily dose for your specific skin tone. If your skin reddens or burns any vitamin D made will be destroyed.

Supplementing with vitamin D drops is also a great way to build up your vitamin D levels, especially if you do not live in a sunny area and/or if you live above the 35th parallel.

As a general rule, on days you are getting your vitamin D from the sun, you do not also need to take your higher dose of oral vitamin D supplement. There is no need to double dose.

How much oral vitamin D should I be taking if I don't have blood work done?

The following doses are taken from the vitamin D experts at the Vitamin D Council (www.vitamindcouncil.org) and are provided as a guideline.

Other factors need to be considered such as where you live (latitude/cloud cover), any illnesses you are fighting and any illnesses or medication that could interfere with vitamin D production. You could require a higher dose (or lower dose if you have kidney or liver problems). As always, on days you are getting adequate sun exposure you do not need to supplement with vitamin D.

On days you are not getting your vitamin D from the sun these doses are a good general guideline:

- Adults: 5,000 IU/day

- Pregnant or lactating: 4-6,000 IU/day

- Breast fed infants: 1,000 IU/day (unless mother is taking 4-6,000 IU/day)

- Formula fed infants: 600 IU/day (formula supplies the other 400 IU/day)

- Children 1-3 years: 2,000 IU/day

- Children over 4-10: 3,000 IU/day

- Children 11 and older: 5,000 IU/day

Is it true that some people don't utilize vitamin D efficiently and must take a higher dose to have the same effect? If so, how can I find out if I have this condition?

Yes, there are some genetic conditions that effect the functioning of vitamin D. This is not something you can diagnosis yourself and must be addressed with your physician, or a physician knowledgeable in VDR genomic abnormalities. Genetic testing is done to evaluate the function of the vitamin D receptor (VDR) and thereby your ability to effectively utilize the active form of vitamin D.

What form of vitamin D is best?

Vitamin D_3. Most vitamin D_3 is able to be absorbed into the body. The major stumbling block is knowing when to take it. It is best absorbed after eating a meal with fats included since it is a fat soluble vitamin.

Is it okay to take while pregnant?

Yes! In fact, it is very important for fetal nervous system development. Make sure you get your levels checked throughout your pregnancy.

Is it a good idea to take vitamin D while nursing?

Yes again! Especially in colder, darker regions of the country like Seattle or Boston. After your baby weans, or goes onto a cup or formula make sure the 'vitamin D' is still optimal for him or her.

What medications interfere with vitamin D levels?

These medications increase the metabolism of vitamin D and may decrease serum 25(OH)D levels:

- Phenytoin (Dilantin)
- Fosphenytoin (Cerebyx)
- Phenobarbital (Luminal)
- Carbamazepine (Tegretol)
- Rifampin (Rimactane)

This is not a comprehensive list and you should consult your doctor regarding medications you are taking and vitamin D supplementation.

Which medications conflict with vitamin D absorption?

Several medications can hamper the absorption of vitamin D. One popular medication that interferes is HCT2 (a water pill).

What if I have a sun allergy?

If you have a sun allergy and need to avoid the sun or cover your skin with clothing when outdoors, please supplement with oral vitamin D to get the tremendous health benefits of vitamin D.

What side effects of vitamin D are there?

It is impossible to get too much vitamin D from the sun. Over exposure to the sun results in sun burn and the destruction of any vitamin D produced.

If you getting too much 'oral' vitamin D you may experience hypercalcemia effects. These are: nausea, vomiting, headaches. If this is prolonged you may die. The toxicity level is between 150 – 200 ng/ml. It is important to note that it is very difficult to reach this toxic level. Monitoring closely every 2-3 months is a good idea. In general, if you are in the summertime sun for a ½ to 1 hour 3-4 times per week without sunscreen, you probably won't require any extra oral vitamin D.

<u>What quantity of vitamin D causes toxic effects on the body?</u>

It isn't the quantity of vitamin D that causes toxicity, but the level of 25(OH)D in your body that indicates toxicity. Quantities in the blood over 150 ng/ml are considered toxic. These levels are extremely hard to obtain as the body regularly uses 25(OH)D in all it's many processes.
Please consult with your physician to regularly monitor your vitamin D 25(OH)D levels to prevent any possibility of intoxication.

<u>What is the effect of vitamin D intoxication?</u>

The development of hypercalcemia which can lead to nephrocalcinosis and coronary sclerosis.

<u>I live in a sunny climate and my religious traditions keep my skin covered. How can I best protect my health and honor my spiritual beliefs?</u>

Whenever anyone can't get their vitamin D from the sunshine, I highly recommend supplementing with oral vitamin D.

<u>I live below the 35th parallel, but I work indoors all the time and only get the afternoon sunshine. Is that enough vitamin D?</u>

No. Afternoon sunlight is not as strong and solar noon sunlight and is not as efficient as synthesizing vitamin D in your skin.   It is likely you will require additional oral vitamin D supplementation if you are not getting solar noon sunlight on your arm, face and legs at least 3-4 times per week.

<u>I'm worried about getting skin cancer. Will supplementing with oral vitamin D be enough?</u>

The short answer is YES. Of course, taking an oral supplement of vitamin D can make up for the sunlight you skin isn't getting. It is also important to know that by exposing your skin to a small amount of sunshine regularly, will actually help protect the skin from skin cancer.

<u>Is it true that vitamin D can be washed off?</u>

Yes. Dr. Cannell, at the Vitamin D Council, has written about this phenomenon in his newsletters, stating that, "washing with soap after being in the sun reduces the amount of vitamin D you get." He explains that the body oils (sebum) which contain vitamin D can be washed off, thereby reducing the overall amount of vitamin D your body gets. As you may remember from Chapter 4, vitamin D is produced in the epidermis, the top layer of the skin, and the process of converting pre-vitamin D to vitamin D takes 3-4 hours to complete. If you have been in the sun, avoid showering with soap for at least 4 hours in order to prevent the vitamin D in the oil glands from being washed off.

Does vitamin D really help with inflammation?

Yes! Vitamin D has a vast and remarkable effect on the entire body. In its active form it controls inflammation. On the reverse side, if you are low or deficient in vitamin D, the inflammatory hormones in the body are activated (interleukins and cytokines) and inflammation occurs. This process is similar to low thyroid and for premenopausal women.

I have fibromyalgia. Will taking vitamin D help with the pain and inflammation I experience?

Fibromyalgia patients can benefit from taking vitamin D. It is however a complicated disease and other considerations need to be monitored by your physician. I recommend getting your baseline serum level checked. Then work with your physician to increase your serum levels until they are between 65-80 ng/ml. Have your levels checked regularly to be sure you are staying optimal.

Is there a test that would show my genetic ability to utilize vitamin D in my body efficiently?

Yes, there are several genetic testing companies that will evaluate the function of the vitamin D receptor. Please visit your physician for guidance and recommendations on whether or not you need genetic testing and possibly a different vitamin D treatment plan.

What medical conditions are particularly at risk for vitamin D deficiency?

Fat malabsorption conditions
Cystic fibrosis
Cholestatic liver
Celiac disease
Whipple's disease
Crohn's disease
By-pass surgery
Obesity
Patients with skin grafts - due to decrease in 7-dehydrocholesterol in the skin
Liver failure (mild to moderate) malabsorption of vitamin D, but production of 25(OH)D is possible.

Liver failure (90% or more) inability to make sufficient 25(OH)D
Nephrotic syndrome – substantial loss of 25(OH)D to urine
Chronic kidney disease
Rickets – heritable disorder
Sarcoidosis
Tuberculosis
Some lymphomas
Hyperparathyroidism – reduces levels of 25(OH)D
Primary hyperparathyroidism – reduces levels of 25(OH)D and increases 1,25(OH)2D
Tumor induced osteomalacia

<u>What medical conditions can be helped with normal serum levels of vitamin D?</u>
Taken from the National Library of Medicine – National Institute of Health's Medline website

Osteomalacia
Psoriasis
Rickets
Familial hypophosphatemia
Fanconi syndrome-related hypophosphatemia
Hyperparathyroidism due to low vitamin D levels
Inflammation
Cancer prevention
Corticosteriod-induced osteoporosis
Anti-convulsant-induced osteomalacia
Osteoporosis
Renal osteodystrophy
Diabetes – (Type I/Type 2)
Fall prevention
Hepatic osteodystrophy
High blood pressure (hypertension)
Hypertriglyceridemia
Multiple Sclerosis
Myelodysplactic syndrome
Osteogenesis imperfect (OI)
Osteoporosis in cystic fibrosis
Prostate Cancer
Proximal myopathy
Seasonal Affective Disorder
Senile warts

Tooth retention
Improved muscle strength

Where in the body is the VDR (vitamin D receptor) found and therefore needed and used?

Zimmerman, A. Vitamin D in preventative medicine: are we ignoring the evidence?

Intestinal cells
Muscle cells
Osteoblasts
Distal rental cells
Parathyroid cells
Islet cells, pancreas
Epidermal cells
Circulating monocytes
Transformed B-cells
Activated T-cells
Neurons
Placenta
Skin fibroblasts
Chondrocytes
Colon enterocytes
Liver cells
Prostate cells
Ovarian cells
Keratinocytes of skin
Endocrine cells, stomach
Aortic epithelial cells
Pituitary cells

What diseases and conditions could be associated with a vitamin D deficiency?

If you have been diagnosed with any of the following diseases or conditions, it is possible that you have a vitamin D deficiency. Please see your physician and request a blood test of your 25(OH)D serum level. 25(OH)D is the circulating form that most accurately measures vitamin D bio-availability. By therapeutically treating vitamin D deficiency and raising your serum levels you will harness the miraculous healing powers of vitamin D.

Asthma
Autism

Bone fractures that are not healing normally or in the time expected
Breast Cancer
Colon Cancer
Lung Cancer
Prostate Cancer
Ovarian Cancer
Chronic pain – non-specific pain disorder
Colitis
Depression
Diabetes – Type I
Fibromyalgia
Heart problems
Hypertension
Influenza (flu)
Infertility
Irritable Bowel Syndrome
Low back pain
Lupus
Macular degeneration
Multiple Sclerosis
Non-degenerative joint disease
Obesity
Osteomalacia
Osteopenia
Osteoporosis
Periodontal disease
Propensity to fall
Psoriasis
Rheumatoid Arthritis
Rickets
Schizophrenia
Seasonal Affective Disorder (SAD)
Skin disorders
Stroke
Transplant patients
Viral infections – (frequent common cold)
Weak Muscles

Am I at risk for being vitamin D deficient?

Anyone who is not getting adequate sunlight exposure most of the year or who is not taking an oral vitamin D supplement to make up for the lack of sunlight is likely low in their vitamin D status.

Those at a particular risk include:
Pregnant
Breastfeeding
Breast fed babies (breast milk is not a sufficient source of vitamin D).
12-18 month olds (weaned from breast milk/formula without supplementing with vitamin D)
Children who don't often play outside and whose parents always put on sunscreen
Adolescents
Over 49
Obese
Vegan
Nursing home residents
House bound individuals
If you rarely spend time in the sun
If you always wear sunscreen
If you live above 40º latitude (see latitude chart for vitamin D production in the skin)
If you do not supplement with vitamin D
If you do not eat vitamin D rich foods (oily fish, liver, egg yolks etc)
If you have dark skin and do not live near the equator

Appendix B: Resources

As a licensed naturopathic physician, specializing in natural therapies, it is very important to me to offer the highest quality vitamin supplements available on the market. Two brands that I regularly use in my practice for vitamin D supplementation are:

Thorne Research
www.thorne.com
1-800-228-1966

and

Biotics Research Corporation
(281)344-0909

Vitamin D Test Kit
The Vitamin D Council now offers an in-home vitamin D test kit for measuring your vitamin D levels. You can purchase this test on the council's website at www.vitamindcouncil.org. This is a great place to get your test kit because a portion of the proceeds goes to support the website and the continuous breadth of information on vitamin D that the researchers provide to the public.

You can find more recommendations for quality supplements suggested in the therapy chapters at my website: www.DrLMesser.com

For more information on vitamin D visit our website at
www.powerfulmedicine-vitD.com.

Appendix C: What do the experts have to say?

The following quotations have been taken from some of the hundreds of research articles published on vitamin D.

<u>General</u>

"Adequate sun exposure is essential for human health."
Kimlin, M. et.al. Location and vitamin D synthesis: Is the hypothesis validated by geographical data?

"One billion people worldwide are vitamin D insufficient."
Prof. Roger Bouillon. University of Leuven.
Kimlin, M. et.al. Location and vitamin D synthesis: Is the hypothesis validated by geographical data?

"Vitamin D deficiency is an unrecognized epidemic in most adults who are not exposed to adequate sunlight."
Holick, MF Evolution and Function of vitamin D

"We must move away from the concept that vitamin D is a vitamin."
DeLuca, H. Overview of general physiologic features and functions of vitamin D

"The insights into the new biological functions of 1,25(OH)2D3 in regulating cell growth, modulating the immune system and modulating the rennin-angiotensin system provides an explanation for why diminished sun exposure at higher latitudes is associated with increased risk of dying of many common cancers, developing type 1 diabetes and multiple sclerosis, and having higher incidence of hypertension."
Holick, MF Evolution and Function of vitamin D

"Evidence is emerging about the protective effects of UV exposure for cancer (breast, colo-rectal, prostate), auto-immune diseases (multiple sclerosis, type II diabetes) and even mental disorders, such as schizophrenia."
Kimlin, M. et.al. Location and vitamin D synthesis: Is the hypothesis validated by geographical data?

"Of great interest is the role it can play in decreasing the risk of many chronic illnesses, including common cancers, autoimmune diseases, infectious diseases and cardiovascular disease."
Holick, M. Vitamin D Deficiency

"Given that sunshine exposure is the most important source of vitamin D, one should expect that vitamin D status depends on geographic location relative to the equator."
Lips, P. et.al. A global study of Vitamin D status and parathyroid function in post-menopausal women with Osteoporosis: baseline data from the multiple outcomes of Raloxifene Evaluation Clinical Trial.

History

In 1936, Dr. Peller, noticed US Navy personnel who experienced an excess of skin cancer, also showed significantly reduced incidence of non-skin cancers. He then advocated deliberately acquiring skin cancer, which is relatively easy to detect and treat, as a form of vaccination against more life threatening and less treatable cancers.
Peller. 1936. Carcinogenesis as a means of reducing cancer mortality. Lancet 2.
Reichrath, J. The challenge resulting from positive and negative effects of sunlight: How much solar UV exposure is appropriate to balance between risks of vitamin D deficiency and skin cancer?

Five years later, in 1941, pathologist, Dr. Frank Apperly, further explained that "the presence of skin cancer is really only an occasional accompaniment of a relative cancer immunity in some way related to exposure to ultraviolet radiation. "A closer study of the action of solar radiation on the body, might well reveal the nature of cancer immunity."
Apperly, FL. The relation of solar radiation to Cancer mortality in North America. (1941)
Reichrath, J. The challenge resulting from positive and negative effects of sunlight: How much solar UV exposure is appropriate to balance between risks of vitamin D deficiency and skin cancer?

Politics

"For more than 50 years, there has been documentation in the medical literature suggesting that regular sun exposure is associated with substantial decreases in death rates from certain cancers and a decrease in overall cancer death rates."
Ainsleigh, H.G. Beneficial Effects of Sun Exposure on Cancer Mortality

Dermatologists and other clinicians have to recognize that there is convincing evidence that the protective effect of less intense solar UV radiation outweighs its mutagenic effects.
Reichrath, J. The challenge resulting from positive and negative effects of sunlight: How much solar UV exposure is appropriate to balance between the risk of vitamin D deficiency and skin cancer?

"Despite these reassuring studies (more than 1,000) the public health and medical communities have not adopted use of vitamin D for cancer prevention. The cost of a daily dose of vitamin D3 (1,000 IU) is less than 5 cents, which could be balanced against the high human and economic costs of treating cancer attributable to insufficiency of vitamin D. Leadership from the public health community will provide the best hope for action."
Garland, C. et.al. The Role of Vitamin D in Cancer Prevention

In fact, current recommendations for vitamin D are not designed to ensure anything. They are simply based on the old, default strategy for setting a nutritional guideline, which is to recommend an amount of nutrient similar to what healthy people are eating.
Vieth, R, and Fraser, D. Vitamin D insufficiency: no recommended dietary allowance exists for this nutrient.

Eventually, an RDA based on objective evidence will replace the current guesstimated AI for vitamin D.
Vieth, R, and Fraser, D. Vitamin D insufficiency: no recommended dietary allowance exists for this nutrient.

"The global burden of UV deficient diseases was estimated for the WHO (World Health Organization) at 3.3 billion life-years annually, almost 2,000 times greater than the BOD (Burden Of Disease) of excessive UV exposure...Adequate UV exposure would alleviate the sizeable burden of vitamin D deficiency."
Kimlin, M. et.al. Location and vitamin D synthesis: Is the hypothesis validated by geographical data?

Cancer

"The evidence suggests that efforts to increase vitamin D status, for example by vitamin D supplementation, could reduce cancer incidence and mortality at low cost, with few or no adverse effects.
Garland, C. et.al. The Role of Vitamin D in Cancer Prevention

"There is compelling epidemiologic observations that suggest that living at higher latitudes is associated with increased risk of many common deadly cancers"
Holick, M. Vitamin D: It's role in cancer prevention and treatment

"The results of the current study demonstrate that much of the geographic variation in cancer mortality rates in the U.S. can be attributed to variation in solar UV-B radiation exposure. Thus, many lives could be extended through increased careful exposure to solar UV-B radiation and more safely, vitamin D_3 supplementation, especially in non summer months."
Grant, W. An estimate of premature cancer mortality in the U.S. due to inadequate doses of solar ultraviolet-B radiation. Cancer 2002;94:1867-75. © American Cancer Society

"The annual number of premature deaths from cancer due to lower UV-B exposures was 21,700 for white Americans, 1,400 for black Americans, and 500 for Asian Americans and other minorities."
Grant, W. An estimate of premature cancer mortality in the U.S. due to inadequate doses of solar ultraviolet-B radiation. Cancer 2002;94:1867-75. © American Cancer Society

Cancer Prevention

"Directly or indirectly, 1,25-dihydroxyvitamin D controls more than 200 genes, including genes responsible for the regulation of cellular proliferation, differentiation, apoptosis, and angiogenesis."
Holick, M. Vitamin D Deficiency

"People living at higher latitudes are at increased risk for Hodgkin's lymphoma as well as colon, pancreatic, prostate, ovarian, breast, and other cancers and are more likely to die from these cancers as compared with people living at lower latitudes."
Holick, M. Vitamin D Deficiency

"It (vitamin D) has widespread effects on cellular differentiation and proliferation, and can modulate immune responsiveness, and central nervous system function. Moreover, accumulating epidemiological and molecular evidence suggests that 1,25-dihydroxyvitaminD_3 acts a chemopreventative agent against several malignancies including cancers of the prostate and colon."
Lin, R., White, J. The pleiotropic actions of vitamin D

Cancer and Season of Diagnosis

"We found evidence of substantial seasonality in cancer survival, with diagnosis in summer and autumn associated with improved survival compared with that in winter, especially in female breast cancer patients and both male and female lung cancer patients." "We also found sunlight exposure to be a predictor of cancer survival."
Hyun-Sook Lim et.al. Cancer survival is dependent on season of diagnosis and sunlight exposure.

Occupational Exposure and Cancer

Occupations with the highest exposure to sunlight are associated with significantly reduced death rates from breast and colon cancer.
Freedman, D.M., et.al. Sunlight and mortality from breast, ovarian, colon, prostate and non-melanoma skin cancer: a composite death certificate based case-control study.

Breast Cancer

"Frequent sun exposure acts to prevent cancers that have death rates from 25-65% with 138,000 fatalities per year."
Ainsleigh, H.G. Beneficial Effects of Sun Exposure on Cancer Mortality

Serum levels of vitamin D (25(OH)D) of at least 52ng/ml had a 50% lower risk of breast cancer than women with levels less than 13ng/ml.
Garland, C. et.al. Vitamin D and prevention of breast cancer: pooled analysis

"In this cohort analysis, we found that high exposure to sunlight was associated with a 25-65% reduction in breast cancer risk among women whose longest residence was in a state of high solar radiation."
John, E. et.al. Vitamin D and Breast Cancer Risk: The NHANES I Epidemiologic Follow-up Study, 1971-1975 to 1992.

Colon Cancer

"Participants in the Women's Health Initiative who at baseline has a 25-hydroxyvitamin D concentration of 12 ng/ml (30 nmol/L) had a 253% increase in the risk of colorectal cancer over the 8 year follow-up period."
Holick, M. Vitamin D Deficiency

"The geographic distribution of colon cancer is similar to the historical geographic distribution of rickets. The highest death rates from colon cancer occur in areas that had the highest prevalence of rickets – regions with winter ultraviolet deficiency, generally due to a combination of high or moderately high latitude, high sulfur content air pollution (acid haze), higher than average stratospheric ozone thickness, and persistently thick winter cloud cover. "
Garland, C., Garland, F., and Gorham, E. Calcium and Vitamin D

"These findings, which are consistent with laboratory results, indicate that most cases of colon cancer may be prevented with regular intake of calcium in the range of 1,800 mg per day, in a dietary context that includes 800IU per day (20ug) of vitamin D_3."
Garland, C., Garland, F., and Gorham, E. Calcium and Vitamin D

Lung Cancer

"While cigarette smoking is the undisputed main cause of lung cancer, there exists an inverse relationship between lung cancer and sunlight exposure. In an ecological study analyzing data from 111 countries, it was found that lung cancer rates were lowest near the equator with an increase in incidence rising the further from the equator. The mechanism is likely the higher serum levels of vitamin D metabolites which show anti-carcinogenic characteristics."
Mohr, SB et al. Could ultraviolet B irradiance and vitamin D be associated with lower incidence of lung cancer?

Ovarian Cancer

"In general, ovarian cancer incidence and mortality is higher in northern than southern latitudes. This ecologic study tests the hypothesis that vitamin D produced in the skin from sunlight exposure may be associated with a protective action in ovarian cancer mortality. —- Conclusion: this ecologic study supports the hypothesis that sunlight may be a protective factor for ovarian cancer mortality."
Lefkowitz, E.S. and Garland, C.F. Sunlight, vitamin D, and ovarian cancer mortality rates in US women.

Prostate Cancer

"Certain risk factors for prostate cancer, including advanced age and African American ethnicity, are associated with reduced vitamin D levels."
Guyton, K. et al. Vitamin D and Vitamin D analogs as cancer chemopreventative agents

Auto-Immune Diseases

"Vitamin D is a member of the steroid thyroid super family of nuclear receptors. Active vitamin D functions by binding to the VDR...All members of the steroid hormone super family have been shown to regulate gene transcription."
Cantorna, M. Vitamin D and its role in immunology: Multiple Sclerosis and inflammatory bowel disease.

Diabetes

"Vitamin D supplementation was also associated with reduced incidence of type I diabetes and with improvement in type II diabetes."
Garland, C. et.al. The Role of Vitamin D in Cancer Prevention

"In Finland, vitamin D supplementation of infants was associated with reduction by 4/5 in incidence of type 1 diabetes."
Garland, C. et.al. The Role of Vitamin D in Cancer Prevention

Multiple Sclerosis

"MS is a disease that is essentially unknown at the equator and the prevalence of the disease increases in populations that live farther away from the equator (Hayes, 2000)."
Cantorna, M. Vitamin D and its role in immunology: Multiple Sclerosis and inflammatory bowel disease.

"A recent, large epidemiological study showed that women with the highest vitamin D intakes (used supplements) had a 40% reduction in the risk of developing MS. (Munger et.al. 2004)"
Cantorna, M. Vitamin D and its role in immunology: Multiple Sclerosis and inflammatory bowel disease.

"Experimental Autoimmune Encephalitis (EAE) is an autoimmune disease believed to be the model for the human disease Multiple Sclerosis." Researching EAE allows an extrapolation of similar results to be made for Multiple Sclerosis. Drs. Cantorna, Hayes and DeLuca's research, published in Immunology, holds significant importance and hope for the prevention and treatment of MS. The research published in 1996 shown that the administration of vitamin D was able to completely prevent the development of EAE. Additionally, when initial symptoms of EAE developed, and vitamin D was administered, the disease was halted. When vitamin D was withheld, and the vitamin D levels were deficient, the disease once again progressed.
Cantorna, M., Hayes, C. and DeLuca, H. 1,25-dihydroxyvitamin D3, reversibly blocks the progression of relapsing encephalomyelitis, a model of multiple sclerosis.

Inflammatory Bowel Disease (IBD) – Crohn's disease and ulceratic colitis

"IBD is most prevalent in northern climates."
Cantorna, M. Vitamin D and its role in immunology: Multiple Sclerosis and inflammatory bowel disease.

"Vitamin D deficiency is common in patients with IBD even when the disease is in remission. It is unclear why vitamin D deficiency occurs more frequently in IBD. It is probably due to the combined effects of low vitamin D intake, malabsorption of many nutrients including vitamin D, and decreased outdoor activities in climates that are not optimal for vitamin D synthesis in the skin."
Cantorna, M. Vitamin D and its role in immunology: Multiple Sclerosis and inflammatory bowel diseases

TB (Tuberculosis)

"According to the World Health Organization (WHO) infections with M.tb. (Tuberculosis) kills a human being every 15 seconds. In 2005 alone, there were estimated to be nearly 2 billion deaths worldwide attributed to TB....TB is the leading cause of death worldwide in women of reproductive age and individuals with HIV. To bring this pandemic closer to home, estimates are that 10-15 million people residing in the United States are infected with M.tb. And, like the situation worldwide, mycobacterium infection is a leading cause of death among patients with AIDS in this country. The concern for the AIDS patients is acute give the recent emergence of extensively drug-resistant (XDR) TB and its high mortality rate...Considering the current coordinate pandemics in vitamin D insufficiency, tuberculosis and AIDS across sub-Saharan Africa and South Asia, simple repair of vitamin D insufficiency in those populations may prove to be effective adjuvant therapy for the immunocompromised host with tuberculosis."
Adams, et.al. Vitamin D in defense of the Human Immune Response

Bone health

"We confirm earlier observations that the presence of vitamin D insufficiency may be a common occurrence in osteopenic/osteoporotic patient populations even in sunlight-enriched, lower latitude environments and demonstrate that return to normal vitamin D balance can result in a prompt and substantial increase in bone mineral density."
Adams, J. et.al. Resolution of vitamin D insufficiency in Osteopenic Patients result in rapid recovery of bone mineral density.

"Vitamin D deficiency leads to secondary hyperparathyroidism, increased bone turnover, and bone loss and, when severe, to osteomalacia."
Lips, P. et.al. A global study of Vitamin D status and parathyroid function in post-menopausal women with Osteoporosis: baseline data from the multiple outcomes of Raloxifene Evaluation Clinical Trial.

"Because osteomalacia is a known cause of persistent, nonspecific musculoskeletal pain, screening all outpatients with such pain for hypovitaminosis D should be standard practice in clinical care."
Plotnikoff, G. et.al. Prevalence of Severe Hypovitaminosis D in patients with persistent, nonspecific musculoskeletal pain.

"Vitamin D deficiency has been implicated as a cause of hip fractures. In addition, vitamin D and calcium supplementation have been demonstrated to decrease the incidence of hip and other nonspine fractures."
Lips, P. et.al. A global study of Vitamin D status and parathyroid function in post-menopausal women with Osteoporosis: baseline data from the multiple outcomes of Raloxifene Evaluation Clinical Trial.

"Of the African American, East African, Hispanic, and American Indian patients, 100% had deficient levels of vitamin D."
Plotnikoff, G. et.al. Prevalence of Severe Hypovitaminosis D in patients with persistent, nonspecific musculoskeletal pain.

Cardiovascular Health

"Published data suggest a linear rise in blood pressure at increasing distances from the equator. Similarly, blood pressure is higher in the winter than summer. Blood pressure also is affected by variations in skin pigmentation."
Rostand, S. Ultraviolet light may contribute to geographic and racial blood pressure differences.

Muscle/Skeletal Pain
Vitamin D deficiency causes muscle weakness
Holick, M. Vitamin D Deficiency

"All patients with persistent, nonspecific musculoskeletal pain are at high risk for the consequences of unrecognized and untreated severe hypovitaminosisD."
Plotnikoff, G. et.al. Prevalence of Severe Hypovitaminosis D in patients with persistent, nonspecific musculoskeletal pain.

Age

"Vitamin D deficiency was present in many US adolescents in this urban clinic-based sample. The prevalence was highest in African American teenagers and during winter, although the problem seems to be common across sex, season and ethnicity."
Gordon, C. et.al. Prevalence of Vitamin D deficiency among healthy adolescents.

"Ageing has been shown to affect vitamin D synthesis primarily through a reduced capacity of skin biosynthesis."
Hill, T. et.al. Vitamin D status of 51-75 year old Irish women: its determinants and impact on biochemical indices of bone turnover.

"The data suggest that the skin thinning that occurs with age lowers the serum 25(OH)D, which presumably could be overcome by greater sunlight exposure. Such a simple change in lifestyle might help to reduce secondary hyper-parathyroidism in the elderly and help stem the rising tide of hip fractures predicted as the world's population ages. Alternatively, a small dose of oral vitamin D given regularly could have the same effect."
Need, A. et al. Vitamin D status: effects on parathyroid hormone and 1,25-dihydroxyvitamin D in postmenopausal women.

Vitamin D insufficiency in healthy adults

"Low vitamin D status was prevalent in these young adults in northern Europe in winter, although the vitamin D intake met the recommendation."
Lambert-Allardt, CJ et.al. Vitamin D deficiency and bone health in healthy adults in Finland: could this be a concern for other parts of Europe?

"The prevalence of hypovitaminosis D was unexpectedly high in this population of non-elderly, non-housebound, primary care outpatients with persistent, nonspecific musculoskeletal pain refractory to standard pharmaceutical agents. Of all patients, 93% had deficient levels of vitamin D."
Plotnikoff, G. et.al. Prevalence of Severe Hypovitaminosis D in patients with persistent, nonspecific musculoskeletal pain.

"The take-home message from Plotnikoff and Quigley's observations is that when patients with non-specific skeleton-muscular pain are evaluated, their serum 25-hydroxyvitamin D levels should be obtained."
Holick, MF Vitamin D Deficiency: What a Pain It Is

Pregnancy and Infants

"The levels of deficiency in women of childbearing age are consistent with increased risk for bearing children with adverse fetal affects or for severe neonatal illnesses."
Plotnikoff, G. et.al. Prevalence of Severe Hypovitaminosis D in patients with persistent, nonspecific musculoskeletal pain.

"Also at risk were pregnant and lactating women who were thought to be immune to vitamin D deficiency since they took a daily prenatal vitamin containing 400 IU of vitamin D. (70% took a prenatal vitamin, 90% ate fish and 93% drank approximately 2.3 glasses of milk per day): 73% of the women and 80% of their infants were vitamin D deficient (25-hydroxyvitamin D level, <20ng per milliliter) at the time of birth."
Holick, M. Vitamin D Deficiency

"Infants who are exclusively breast fed and do not receive vitamin D supplementation are at high risk of vitamin D deficiency, particularly if they have dark skin and/or receive little sun exposure. Human milk generally provides 25 IU of vitamin D per liter, which is not enough for an infant if it is the sole source of vitamin D."
Linus Pauling Institute. Oregon State University

"Ensuring adequate vitamin D supplementation for infants could help reverse the increasing trend in the incidence of type 1 diabetes."
Hypponen, E. Intake of vitamin D and risk of type 1 diabetes: a birth-cohort study

Dosing

"To offer some perspective here, an adult with white skin, exposed to summer sunshine while wearing a bathing suit, generates about 250 ug (10,000 IU) of vitamin D3 in 15-20 minutes; longer exposure generates no more vitamin D."
Vieth, R and Fraser D. Vitamin D insufficiency: no recommended dietary allowance existed for this nutrient.

"Currently, most experts in the field believe that intakes of between 1,000 to 4,000 IU will lead to a more healthy serum 25(OH)D, in the range of 75 nmol/L that will offer significant protect effects against cancers of the breast, colon, prostate, ovary, lungs and pancreas."
Ingraham, B.A. et.al. Molecular basis of the potential of vitamin D to prevent cancer.

"Heaney et.al. estimated that the body uses 3,000 to 5,000 IU per day of vita-min D."
Holick MF Vitamin D deficiency: What a pain it is

"Current estimations for an adequate oral intake are obviously much too low to achieve an optimal vitamin D status and thus to effectively prevent chronic vitamin D-dependent diseases."
Zimmerman, A. Vitamin D in preventative medicine: are we ignoring the evidence?

"The major sources of vitamin D for most humans are casual exposure of the skin to solar ultraviolet B (UVB; 290-315 nm) radiation and from dietary intake."
Chen, T. et.al. Factors that influence the cutaneous synthesis and dietary sources of vitamin D

"The cutaneous synthesis of vitamin D is a function of skin pigmentation and of the solar zenith angle which depends on latitude, season and time of day."
Chen, T. et.al. Factors that influence the cutaneous synthesis and dietary sources of vitamin D

Vitamin D intoxication

"There are no reports of vitamin D intoxication in healthy adults after intensive sunlight exposure."
Zimmerman, A. Vitamin D in preventative medicine: are we ignoring the evidence?

In all cases of vitamin D intoxication 25(OH)D levels were clearly above 200nmol/L. Levels of up to 1,000nmol/L and more have been observed.
Zimmerman, A. Vitamin D in preventative medicine: are we ignoring the evidence?

"In adults, vitamin D intoxication has been observed after the administration of very high therapeutic doses (1978), in association with an over-the-counter supplement that contained 26 to 430 times the vitamin D3 amount listed by the manufacturer (2001), and in association with an accidentally excessive overfortification of consumers' milk with vitamin D3."
Zimmerman, A. Vitamin D in preventative medicine: are we ignoring the evidence?

Food Sources

"49% of 173 milk samples collected in the United States and British Columbia, Canada, contained less than 80% of the vitamin D content on the label and 14% did not contain any detectable vitamin D, raising a serious question about the role of milk in providing the consumers with their vitamin D requirement."
Chen, T. et.al. Factors that influence the cutaneous synthesis and dietary sources of vitamin D

"It is believed that oily fish such as salmon, mackerel and bluefish are excellent sources of vitamin D3. However, our analysis of the vitamin D content in a variety of fish species indicates that farmed salmon, the most widely consumed fish in the US, contained about one quarter of the vitamin D3 found in wild caught salmon from Alaska."
Chen, T. et.al. Factors that influence the cutaneous synthesis and dietary sources of vitamin D

"There needs to be a reevaluation of the vitamin D content in all fish and other foods that have been traditionally recommended as good sources of naturally occurring vitamin D."
Chen, T. et.al. Factors that influence the cutaneous synthesis and dietary sources of vitamin D

"Dietary intake and artificial fortification of foods is a trivial and ineffectual proportion of vitamin D intake for most populations. Adequate UV exposure would alleviate the sizeable burden of vitamin D deficiency."
Kimlin, M. et.al. Location and vitamin D synthesis: Is the hypothsis validated by geophysical data?

Sunscreen

"Application of a sunscreen with sun protection factor 8 reduces the capacity of the skin to produce vitamin D by 95%."
Holick, MF Vitamin D Deficiency: What a Pain It Is

"There is support in the medical literature to suggest that the 17% increase in breast cancer incidence during the 1991-1992 year may be the result of the past decade of pervasive anti-sun advisories from respected authorities, coinciding with effective sunscreen availability. "
Ainsleigh, H.G. Beneficial Effects of Sun Exposure on Cancer Mortality

"In addition, the effectiveness of cutaneous synthesis of vitamin D3 is also determined by the skin pigmentation, because melanin efficiently absorbs UVB radiation."
Chen, T. et.al. Factors that influence the cutaneous synthesis and dietary sources of vitamin D

Clothing

"Even light white cotton, plain weave cloth prevents vitamin D photosynthesis in Caucacians, and the effect persists after exposure to the extraordinary high dose of six MEDs of UV-B radiation."
Matsuoka, L. et.al. Clothing prevents Ultraviolet-B Radiation-Dependent photosynthesis of vitamin D3.

"A detrimental consequence of the UV-B-screening effect of clothing is the interference with vitamin D3 formation and, potentially calcium and bone metabolism."
Matsuoka, L. et.al. Clothing prevents Ultraviolet-B Radiation-Dependent photosynthesis of vitamin D3.

"However, even in the sunniest areas, vitamin D deficiency is common when most of the skin is shielded from the sun. In studies in Saudi Arabia, the United Arab Emirates, Australia, Turkey, India, and Lebanon, 30-50% of children and adults had 25-hydroxyvitamin D levels under 20 ng per milliliter."
Holick, M. Vitamin D Deficiency

"Protection from sunlight by extensive coverage with clothing has also resulted in the production of overt osteomalacia and/or rickets in Bedouins in the Negev Desert (Isreal) and in American Muslims."
Matsuoka, L. et.al. Clothing prevents Ultraviolet-B Radiation-Dependent photosynthesis of vitamin D3.

Skin

"A reduced efficiency of vitamin D3 photosynthesis may partially explain some of the interracial and intraracial differences in vitamin D metabolites and PTH concentrations and the apparent direct association between BP (blood pressure) and the degree of skin pigmentation in African Americans."
Rostand, S. Ultraviolet light may contribute to geographic and racial blood pressure differences.

Vitamin D Winter

"Human skin or [3 alpha-3H]7-dehydrocholesterol exposed to sunlight on cloudless days in Boston (42.2 degrees N) from November through February produced no previtamin D3. In Edmonton (52 degrees N) this ineffective winter period extended from October through March. Further South (34 degrees N and 18 degrees N), sunlight effectively photoconverted 7-dehydroxycholesterol to previtamin D3 in the middle of winter."

Webb, Kline and Holick. Influences of season and latitude on the cutaneous synthesis of vitamin D3: exposure to winter sunlight in Boston and Edmonton will not promote vitamin D3 synthesis in human skin.

Appendix D: References

Analogues

Agoston, E.S. et.al. Vitamin D analogs as anti-carcinogenic agents. Anticancer Agents Med Chem. Jan 2006. 6:1 pp. 53-71.

Dalhoff, K. et.al. A phase II study of the vitamin D analogue Seocalcitol in patients with inoperable hepatocellular carcinoma. British Journal of Cancer. 2003. 89 pp. 252-257.

Griffin, M., Xing, N., Kumar., R. Vitamin D and its Analogs as Regulators of Immune Activation and Antigen Presentation. Annu. Rev. Nutr. 2003. 23:117-145.

Guyton, K. et.al. Vitamin D and vitamin D analogs as cancer chemopreventative agents. Nutrition Reviews. July 2003, 61:7, pp. 227-238.

Guyton, KZ et.al. Cancer chemoprevention using natural vitamin D and synthetic analogs. Annu Rev Pharmacology Toxicol. 2001. 41 pp. 421-442.

Holick, M. Vit D: It's role in cancer prevention and treatment. Progress in Biophysics and Molecular Biology. Sept 2006, 92:1, pp. 49-59

Autism

Almeras, L., Eyles, D. et.al. Developmental vitamin D deficiency alters brain protein expression in the adult rat: implications for neuropsychiatric disorders. Proteomics. 2007. 7, pp. 769-780.

Cui, X., McGrath, J. et.al. Maternal vitamin D depletion alters neurogenesis in the developing rat brain. International Journal of Developmental Neuroscience. 2007. 25(4), pp. 227-232.

Fernandez de Abreu, DA, Eyles, D and Feron, F. Vitamin D, a neuro-immunomodulator: Implications for neurodegenerative and autoimmune diseases. Psychoneuroendocrinology. Jun 20 2009.

Kalueff, A. et.al. Behavioural anomalies in mice evoked by "Tokyo" disruption of the vitamin D receptor. Neuroscience Research. April 2006. 54(4). pp. 254-260.

Auto-immune diseases

(M.S., Rheumatoid Arthritis, Lupus, Diabetes, Fibromyalgia)

Cantorna, M. Vitamin D and its role in immunology: Multiple Sclerosis, and inflammatory bowel disease. Progress in Biophysics and Molecular Biology. Sept. 2006. 92:1 pp. 60-64

Cantorna, M. et.al. 1,25-dihydroxyvitamin D3, reversibly blocks the progression of relapsing encephalymyelitis, a model of multiple sclerosis. Immunology. July 1996. 93:15 pp. 7861-7864.

DeLuca, H, Cantorna, M. Vitamin D: its role and uses in immunology1 FASEB J. 15, 2579-2585 (2001)

Hernan, M. et.al. Geographic variation of MS incidence in two prospective studies of US women. Neurology. 1999. 53 pp 1711-

Hypponen, E. et.al. Intake of vitamin D and risk of type 1 diabetes: a birth-cohort study. The Lancet. Nov 2001. 3:358(9292) pp. 1500-1503.

Munger, K.L. et.al. Vitamin D intake and incidence of multiple sclerosis. Neurology. Jan 2004, 62:1, pp. 60-65.

Pittas, A. et.al. Review: The role of vitamin D and calcium in Type-2 diabetes. A systemic review and meta-analysis. Journal of Clinical Endocrinology and Metabolism. 2007, 92:6, pp. 2017-2029.

Zhang, S.M. et.al. Intakes of carotenoids, vitamin C, and vitamin E and MS risk among two large cohorts of women. Neurology. 2001. 57 pp. 75-80.

Cancer

(Breast, Colon, Lung, Prostate, Ovarian)

Ainsleigh, H.G. Beneficial effects of sun exposure on cancer mortality. Preventative Medicine. Jan 1993. 22:1 pp. 132-140.

Bertone-Johnson, E. et.al. Plasma 25-Hydroxyvitamin D and 1,25-dihydroxyvitamin D and risk of breast cancer. Cancer Epidemiology Biomarkers Prev. Aug. 2005, 14:8 pp. 1991-1997.

Freedman, D.M. et.al. Sunlight and mortality from breast, ovarian, colon, prostrate, and non-melanoma skin cancer: a composite death certificate based case-control study. Occupational and Environmental Medicine. 2002. 59 pp. 257-262.

Garland, C et.al. Vitamin D and prevention of breast cancer: Pooled analysis J. Steroid Biochemistry and Molecular Biology, March 2007, 103:3-5, pp. 708-711

Garland, C. et.al. Geographic variation in breast cancer mortality in the United States: A hypothesis involving exposure to solar radiation. Preventative Medicine. Nov. 1990. 19:6 pp. 614-622.

Garland, C., et.al. The role of vitamin D in cancer prevention. Am. J. Public Health. Feb. 2006, 96:2 pp. 252-261.

Garland, C. Calcium and Vitamin D. Their potential roles in colon and breast cancer prevention. Annals NY Acad Sci. pp.107-119. (need year)

Giovannucci, E. The epidemiology of vitamin D and cancer incidence and mortality: a review (United States). Cancer Causes Control. March 2005. 16:2 pp. 83-95.

Giovannucci, E., Liu, Y, Willett, W.C. Cancer Incidence and Mortality and Vitamin D in Black and White Health Professionals. Cancer Epidemiology Biomarkers & Prevention. Vol. 15 No.12 pp. 2467-2472. (in personal factors section)

Grant, W. An estimate of premature cancer mortality in the U.S. due to inadequate doses of solar ultraviolet-B radiation. American Cancer Society. 2002. 94:6 pp. 1867-1875.

Grant, W. An Ecologic study of dietary and solar ultraviolet-B links to breast carcinoma mortality rates. Am. Cancer Society. 2002. pp. 272-281.

Guyton, K.Z and Kensler, T.W. Prevention of liver cancer. Curr Oncol Rep. Nov 2002. 4:6 pp. 464-470.

Guyton, KZ et.al. Cancer chemoprevention using natural vitamin D and synthetic analogs. Annu Rev Pharmacology Toxicol. 2001. 41 pp. 421-442.

Holick, M.F. Vitamin D: Importance in the prevention of cancers, type 1 diabetes, heart disease, and osteoporosis. American Journal of Clinical Nutrition. March 2004. 79:3 pp. 362-371.

Holick, M. Vit D: It's role in cancer prevention and treatment. Progress in Biophysics and Molecular Biology. Sept 2006, 92:1, pp. 49-59

Holt, P. et.al. Colonic epitheial cell proliferation decreases with increasing levels of serum 25-hydroxy vitamin D. Cancer Epidemiology, Biomarkers & Prevention. January 2202. Vol 11. pp. 113-119.

Ingraham, BA et.al. Molecular basis of the potential of vitamin D to prevent cancer. Curr Med Res Opin. Nov 2007.

Janowsky, E.E. et.al. Association between low levels of 1,25-dihydroxyvitamin D and breast cancer risk. Public Health Nutrition. 1999. 2:3 pp 283-291.

John, E.M. et.al. Vitamin D and breast cancer risk: The NHANES I epidemiologic follow-up study, 1971-1975 to 1992. Cancer Epidemiology Biomarkers and Prevention. May 1999. 8:5 pp. 399-406.

Lefkowitz, E.S. and Garland, C. Sunlight, vitamin D, and ovarian cancer mortality rates in US women. International Journal of Epidemiology. 1994. 23:6 pp. 1133-1136.

Lim, H.S. et.al. Cancer survival is dependent on season of diagnosis and sunlight exposure. Internation Journal of Cancer. 2006. 119 pp. 1530-1536.

Lin, R., White, J. The pleiotropic actions of vitamin D. Bioessays. 2003, 26; pp. 21-28.

Mohr, SB., Garland, C. Could ultraviolet B irradiance and vitamin D be associated with lower incidence rates of lung cancer? J. Epidemiology and Community Health, 2008;62, pp.69-74

Schneider Lefkowitz, E and Garland, C. Sunlight, vitamin D, and ovarian cancer mortality rates in US women. International Journal of Epidemiology. 1994. 23:6 pp. 1133-1136.

Cardiovascular health

Holick, M.F. Vitamin D: Importance in the prevention of cancers, type 1 diabetes, heart disease, and osteoporosis. American Journal of Clinical Nutrition. March 2004. 79:3 pp. 362-371.

Rostand, S. Ultraviolet light may contribute to geographic and racial blood pressure differences. American Heart Association Inc. 1997. 30:2, pp. 150-156. (personal factors)

Zittermann, A. et.al. Putting cardiovascular disease and vitamin D insufficiency into prospective. British Journal of Nutrition. 2005, 94: pp. 483-492.

Depression and Mental Illness

(Non-seasonal, SAD, Schizophrenia)

Alberque, C. and Eytan, A. Chronic pain presenting as major depression in a cross-cultural setting. Int'l Journal Psychiatry in Medicine. 2001, 31:1 pp. 73-76.

NAMI – National Alliance on Mental Illness - http://www.nami.org/content/contentgroups/helpline1/seasonal_affective_disorder(SAD).htm

Seasonal Affective Disorder Association – http://www.sada.org

Mayo Clinic – http://www.mayoclinic.com/health/seasonal-affective-disorder/DS00195

Dosing

Cannell, J. and Hollis, B. Use of Vitamin D in Clinical Practice. Alternative Medicine Review. 2008. 13(1) pp. 6-20.

Glerup, H., Mikkelsen, K. et.al. Commonly recommended daily intake of vitamin D is not sufficient if sunlight exposure is limited. Journal of Internal Medicine. 2000, 247 pp. 260-268.

Goussous, R. et.al. Lack of Effect of Calcium Intake on the 25-hydroxyvitamin D response to Oral Vitamin D3. Journal of Clinical Endocrinology & Metabolism. 2005. 90(2) pp. 707-711.

Grant, W.B. and Holick, M.F. Benefits and requirements of vitamin D for optimal health: A review. Alternative Medicine Review. June 2005. 10:2 pp. 94-111.

Lamberg-Allardt, C. Vitamin D in foods and as supplements. Progress in Biophysics and Molecular Biology. Sept 2006. 92:1 pp. 33-38.

Reichrath, J. The challenge resulting from positive and negative effects of sunlight: How much solar UV exposure is appropriate to balance between risks of vitamin D deficiency and skin cancer? Progress in Biophysics and Molecular Biology. Sept. 2006. 92:1 pp. 9-16.

Vieth, R. et.al. The Urgent need to recommend an intake of vitamin D that is effective. American Journal of Clinical Nutrition 2007. 85 pp. 649-650.

Environmental Factors

(Latitude, Cloud Cover, Air Pollution, Ozone, SZA)

Brustad, M. et.al. Seasonality of UV-radiation and vitamin D status at 69 degrees north. The Royal Society of Chemistry – Photochemical & Photobiological Sciences, 2007. 6 pp.903-908.

Chen, T. et.al. Factors that influence the cutaneous synthesis and dietary sources of vitamin D. Biochemistry and Biophysics. April 2007. 460:2 pp. 213-217.

Kimlin, M. et.al. Location and vitamin D synthesis: Is the hypothesis validated by geophysical data? Journal of Photochemistry and Photobiology B: Biology. March 2007. 86:3 pp. 234-239.

Lubin D. et.al. Global surface ultraviolet radiation climatology from TOMS and ERBE data. Journal of Geophysical Research. 1998. 103:D20 pp. 26,061-26,092.

Webb, A.R. et.al. Influences of season and latitude on the cutaneous synthesis of vitamin D3: exposure to winter sunlight in Boston and Edmonton will not promote vitamin D3 synthesis in human skin. Journal of Clinical Endocrinology and Metabolism. 1988. 67 pp. 373-378.

Webb, A. Who, what, where and when – influences on cutaneous vitamin D synthesis. Progress in Biophysics and Molecular Biology. Sept 2006. 92:1 pp. 17-25.

Immune System

Adams, J. et.al. Vitamin D in defense of the human immune response. Ann. NY Acad. Sci. 2007, 1117. pp. 94-105.

DeLuca, H, Cantorna, M. Vitamin D: its role and uses in immunology1 FASEB J. 15, 2579-2585 (2001) (auto-immune)

Muscular Skeletal

(Osteoporosis, Osteopenia, Osteomalacia, Rheumatology)

Adams. J et.al. Resolution of Vitamin D insufficiency inosteopenic patients result in rapid recovery of bone mineral density. Journal of Clinical Endocrinology & Metabolism. 1999, 84:8 pp. 2729-2730.

Bikle, DD. Role of vitamin D, its metabolites, and analogs in the management of osteoporosis. Rheum Dis Clin North Am. Aug 1994. 20:3 pp. 759-775.

Dawson-Hughes, B. et.al. Effects of calcium and vitamin D supplementation on bone density in men and women 65 years of age or older. The New England Journal of Medicine. Sept. 1997. pp. 670- 676.

Hill, T.R., et.al. Vitamin D status of 51-75 year old Irish women: its determinants and impact on biochemical indices of bone turnover. The Nutrition Society. April 2006, 9:2, pp. 225-233.

Holick, M.F. Vitamin D: Importance in the prevention of cancers, type 1 diabetes, heart disease, and osteoporosis. American Journal of Clinical Nutrition. March 2004. 79:3 pp. 362-371.

Lamberg-Allardt, C.J. et.al. Vitamin D deficiency and bone health in healthy adults in Finland: could this be a concern in other parts of Europe? J Bone Mineral Res. Nov 2001. 16:11 pp. 2066-2073.

Lips, P. et.al. A global study of vitamin D status and parathyroid function in postmenopausal women with osteoporosis: baseline data from the multiple outcomes of raloxifene evaluation clinical trial. Journal of Clinical Endocrinology and Metabolism. 2001. 86:3, pp. 1212-1221.

Plotnikoff, G and Quigley, J. Prevalence of Severe Hypovitaminosis D in patients with Persistent, Non-specific musculoskeletal pain. Mayo Clinic Proceedings; Dec 2003; 78,1463-1470

Personal Factors

(Skin tone, clothing, age, weight, etc)

Chen, T. et.al. Factors that influence the cutaneous synthesis and dietary sources of vitamin D. Biochemistry and Biophysics. April 2007. 460:2 pp. 213-217.

Giovannucci, E., Liu, Y, Willett, W.C. Cancer Incidence and Mortality and Vitamin D in Black and White Health Professionals. Cancer Epidemiology Biomarkers & Prevention. Vol. 15 No.12 pp. 2467-2472.

Looker, A.C. et.al. Serum 25-hydroxyvitamin D status of adolescents and adults in two seasonal subpopulations from NHANES III. Bone. May 2002. 30:5 pp. 771-777.

Matsuoka, L.Y. et.al. Clothing prevents ultraviolet-B radiation-dependent photosynthesis of vitamin D3. Journal of Clinical Endocrinology and Metabolism. 1992. 75:4 pp. 1099-1103.

Need, A. et.al. Vitamin D status: effects on parathyroid hormone and 1,25-dihydroxyvitamin D in postmenopausal women. Am. Journal of Clinical Nutrition. 2000, 71; pp. 1577-1581.

Rostand, S. Ultraviolet light may contribute to geographic and racial blood pressure differences. American Heart Association Inc. 1997. 30:2, pp. 150-156.

Webb, A. Who, what, where and when – influences on cutaneous vitamin D synthesis. Progress in Biophysics and Molecular Biology. Sept 2006. 92:1 pp. 17-25.

Vitamin D needed for Breast Fed Babies: Reference article: Journal of Pediactrics. August 2000. 137 pp. 153-157. http://www.mercola.com

Physiology: General function of vitamin D in the body

Cantorna, M.T. et.al. 1,25-dihydroxyvitamin D cholecalciferol prevents and ameliorates symptoms of experimental murine inflammatory bowel disease. J Nutrition. 2000. 130; pp. 2648-2652.

Cantorna, M.T. et.al. 1,25-dihydroxyvitamin D prevents and ameliorates symptoms in two experiemental models of human arthritis. J Nutrition. 1998. 128; pp. 68-72.

DeLuca, H.F. and Zierold, C. Mechanisms and functions of vitamin D. Nutritional Review. Feb 1998. 56:2 pt 2 pp. S4-S10: discussion S 54-75.

DeLuca, H. Overview of general physiologic features and functions of vitamin D. Am. J. Clin. Nutr. Dec. 2004. 80:6, 1689S-1696S.

Heaney, R. Long-latency deficiency disease: insights from calcium and vitamin D. Am. J. Clin. Nutr. Nov. 2003, 78:5, pp. 912-919.

Holick, M. and Jenkins M. The UV Advantage – The Medical Breakthrough That Shows How to Harness the Power of the Sun for your Health. New York, NY. Ibooks. 2003.

Holick, M. Vitamin D Deficiency. New England Journal of Medicine. July 19th, 2007. 357:3, pp. 266-281.

Hullett, DA, Cantorna MT, et.al. Prolongation of allograft survival by 1,25-dihydroxyvitamin D_3. Transplantation. Oct 1998. 15;66(7) pp. 824-828.

Lemire, JM and Archer, DC. 1,25-dihydroxyvitamin D_3 prevents the in-vivo induction of murine experimental autoimmune encephalitits. J Clin Invest. 1991. 87, pp. 1103-1107.

Lemire, JM. et.al. 1,25-dihydroxyvitamin D_3 attenuated the expression of experimental murine Lupus of MRL/1 mice. AutoImmunity. 1992. 12, pp. 143-148.

Linus Pauling Institute at Oregon State – Micronutrient Research for Optimum Health. Vitamin D - http://lpi.oregonstate.edu/infocenter/vitamins/vitaminD/

Lips, P. Vitamin D physiology. Progress in Biophysics and Molecular Biology. Sept 2006. 92:1 pp. 4-8.

Reichrath, J. The challenge resulting from positive and negative effects of sunlight: How much solar UV exposure is appropriate to balance between risks of vitamin D deficiency and skin cancer? Progress in Biophysics and Molecular Biology. Sept. 2006. 92:1 pp. 9-16.

Zella, JB and DeLuca, HF. Vitamin D and autoimmune diabetes. J Cellular Biology. Feb 2003. 1;88(2) pp. 216-222.

Politics

Hathcock, JN et.al. Risk Assessment for vitamin D. Am J Clinical Nutrition. Jan 2007. 85(1) pp. 6-18.

Vieth, R. et.al. The Urgent need to recommend an intake of vitamin D that is effective. American Journal of Clinical Nutrition 2007. 85 pp. 649-650. (dosing)

Vieth, R. and Fraser, D. Vitamin D insufficiency: no recommended dietary allowance exists for this nutrient. CMAJ June 11, 2002. 116(12) pp.1541-1542

Zittermann, A. Vitamin D in preventative medicine: are we ignoring the evidence? British Journal of Nutrition. 2003, 89: pp. 552-572.

http://www.nlm.nih.gov/medlineplus/druginfo/natural/patient-vitamind.html

RDAs and Safe Upper Levels: Solid Science versus Bureaucratic Bias - http://www.supplementquality.com/news/science-vs-bias1.html.

ODS 2007 Vitamin D Conference (ODS = Office of Dietary Supplements. NIH = National Institute of Health). http://vitamindandhealth.od.nih.gov/

RDAs of vitamin D far too low. Reference Artricle: American Journal of Clinical Nutrition. January 2003. 77:204-210. http://www.mercola.com

http://grants.nih.gov/grants/guide/description.htm

AHRQ Evidence Reports. 158. Effectiveness and Safety of Vitamin D in Relation to Bone Health. http://www.ncbi.nlm.nig.gov/books/

Sunshine Vitamin may ward off breast cancer. Higher levels of vitamin D offer range of health benefits, studies suggest. May 11th, 2006. MSNBC News Services

http://www.msnbc.msn.com/id/12157671/

Vitamin D may fight breast cancer. March 23rd, 2004.

http://newsvote.bbc.co.uk/mpapps/pagetools/print/news.bbc.co.uk/1/hi/health/3558641.stm

Skin Cancer

Alan, M and Rather D. Cutaneous squamous-cell carcinoma. New England J Medicine. 2001. 344, pp. 975-983.

Berwick, M., Armstrong, BK., Ben-Porat, L., et.al. Sun exposure and mortality from melanoma. J Natl Cancer Institute. 2005. 97(3) pp. 193-199.

Elwood, JM and Jopson J. Melanoma and Sun Exposure: An overview of published studies. Int J Cancer. 1997. Oct 9: 73(2). pp. 198-203.

Freedman, D.M. et.al. Sunlight and mortality from breast, ovarian, colon, prostrate, and non-melanoma skin cancer: a composite death certificate based case-control study. Occupational and Environmental Medicine. 2002. 59 pp. 257-262.

Frost, CA and Green, AC. Epidemiology of solar keratoses. Br J Dermatology. 1994. 131, pp. 445-464.

Green, A and Battistutta, D. Incidence and determinates of skin cancer in a high risk Australian population. Int J Cancer. 1990. 46(90) pp. 356-361.

Green, A and Siskind, V. Geographical distribution of cutaneous melanoma in Queensland. Med J Australia. 1983. 1, pp. 407-410.

Osterlind, MA, Tucker, BJ, Stone and OM Jensen. The Danish control study of cutaneous malignant melanoma; Importance of UV light exposure. Int. J Cancer. 1988. 42, pp. 319-324.

Reichrath, J. The challenge resulting from positive and negative effects of sunlight: How much solar UV exposure is appropriate to balance between risks of vitamin D deficiency and skin cancer? Progress in Biophysics and Molecular Biology. Sept. 2006. 92:1 pp. 9-16.

Skin Cancer Foundation - http://www.skincancer.org

Westerdahl, J., Olsson, H., Mosback A., et.al. Is the use of sunscreen a risk factor for melanoma? Melanoma Res. 1995. pp. 59-65.

Vitamin D3 or vitamin D2

Armas, L., Hollis, B. and Heaney, R. Vitamin D2 is much less effective than vitamin D3 in humans. Journal of Clinical Endocrinology and Metabolism. 89:11, pp. 5387-5391.

Trang, H. et.al. Evidence that vitamin D3 increases serum 25-hydroxyvitamin D more efficiently than does vitamin D2. American Journal of Clinical Nutrition. 1998, 68, pp. 854-858.

Sunscreen

Matsuoka, L.Y. et.al. Sunscreens suppress cutaneous vitamin D3 synthesis. Journal of Clinical Endocrinology and Metabolism. 1987. 64 pp. 1165-1168.

Environmental Working Group www.ewg.org

Vitamin D Deficiency

Binkley, N. et.al. Low vitamin D status despite abundant sun exposure. Journal of Clinical Endocrinology and Metabolism. Jun 2007. 92:6 pp. 2130-2135.

Chapuy, M.C., et.al. Prevalence of vitamin D insufficiency in an adult normal population. Osteoporosis International. 1997. 7 pp. 439-443.

Gonzales, G et.al. High prevalence of vitamin D deficiency in Chilean healthy postmenopausal women with normal sun exposure: additional evidence for a worldwide concern. Menopause. May-Jun 2007. 14:3 pt 1 pp. 455-461.

Gordon, C. et.al. Prevalence of vitamin D deficiency among healthy adolescents. Pediatrics and Adolescent Medicine. June 2004. 158:6 pp. 531-537.

Grant, W. Epidemiology of disease risks in relation to vitamin D insufficiency. Progress in Biophysics and Molecular Biology. Sept 2006, 92:1 pp. 65-79.

Holick, M.F. Evolution and function of vitamin D. Recent results Cancer Res. 2003. 164 pp. 3-28.

Holick, M. Vitamin D deficiency: What a pain it is. Mayo Clinic Proceedings. Dec. 2003, 78:12, pp. 1457-1459.

Lips, P. Vitamin D deficiency and secondary hyperparathyroidism in the elderly: consequences for bone loss and fractures and therapeutic implications. Endocrine Reviews. 2001, 22:4, pp. 477-501.

Malabanan, A. Redefining vitamin D insufficiency. The Lancet. March 1998. 351:9105 pp. 805-806.

Rucker, D. et.al. Vitamin D insufficiency in a population of healthy western Canadians. Canadian Medical Association Journal. June 2002. 166:12, pp. 1517-1524.

Zittermann, A. Vitamin D in preventative medicine: are we ignoring the evidence? British Journal of Nutrition. 2003, 89: pp. 552-572.